PSYCHOLOGY PRACTI

EDIT

Arnold P. Goldstein, Syracuse University
Leonard Krasner, Stanford University & SUNY at Stony Brook
Sol L. Garfield, Washington University in St. Louis

PSYCHOLOGICAL TREATMENT
OF CANCER PATIENTS

Titles of Related Interest

PSYCHOLOGICAL TREATMENT OF CANCER PATIENTS
A Cognitive-Behavioral Approach

WILLIAM L. GOLDEN
Cornell Medical College,
Institute for Rational-Emotive Therapy and
Institute for Behavior Therapy

WAYNE D. GERSH
Westchester Center for Behavior Therapy

DAVID M. ROBBINS
Westchester Center for Behavior Therapy

Allyn and Bacon
Boston • London • Toronto • Sydney • Tokyo • Singapore

ISBN 0-205-14551-5

Printed in the United States of America

98 97 96 95 94 93 92   10 9 8 7 6 5 4 3

Library of Congress Catologing-in-Publication Data

Golden, William L.
  Psychological treatment of cancer patients : a cognitive
-behavioral approach / by William L. Golden, Wayne D. Gersh,
David M. Robbins.
    p. cm. -- (Psychology practitioner guidebooks)
  Includes bibliographical references.
  Includes index.

  1. Cancer--Psychological aspects. 2. Cognitive therapy.
3. Cancer--Patients--Rehabilitation. I. Gersh, Wayne D.
II. Robbins, David M. III. Title. IV. Series.
  [DNLM: 1. Cognitive Therapy. 2. Neoplasms--psychology.
3. Neoplasms--therapy. QZ 266 G618p]
RC271.P79G65   1991
616.99'4'0019--dc20
DNLM/DLC
for Library of Congress   90-14367
                                                      CIP

We dedicate this book to:
Tara Lynn Schadlow,
Gertrude Gilson,
and
Ben Gelfand
who died of cancer and touched our lives,

and wish to thank our wives:
Carolyn McCarthy-Golden,
Barbara Gersh,
and
Helene Robbins
for their support and patience
throughout this project

Contents

Preface

As a result of the disease and the invasive medical procedures used to diagnose and treat it, cancer patients are confronted with the possibility of depression, pain, anxiety, phobic reactions, stress-related disorders, sexual and marital difficulties, as well as child management and other family difficulties. We have found that cognitive-behavior therapy can be successfully applied in treating these problems. More and more reports and clinical studies are appearing in the literature indicating that other professionals are getting similar results.

Our decision to write this book grew out of our enthusiasm about the results we have been obtaining with cognitive-behavior therapy. Our goal was to organize and present the various cognitive-behavioral strategies that we have found to be effective in treating cancer patients and to guide the reader in their application. Because of space limitations, we have not been able to discuss every aspect and application of our work. Nevertheless, we have attempted to be as comprehensive as possible and to provide the important details, so that other professionals will be able to apply cognitive-behavioral methods in their work with cancer patients.

Chapter 1

Introduction

The purpose of this book is to guide the reader in the application of cognitive-behavioral methods in the treatment of cancer patients. It is written primarily for those providing psychological treatment and counseling to cancer patients. However, it will also be of interest to individuals involved in providing medical as well as other types of care to these patients. Each technique is described in detail and is broken down into specific steps. Transcripts and case examples are provided for the purpose of demonstrating the application of each procedure.

Although it is written from a cognitive-behavioral perspective, clinicians from other psychotherapeutic orientations will find many of the concepts and techniques useful. Our emphasis here is on the practical application of cognitive-behavioral interventions, and not on theory. Our view is that clinicians from diverse theoretical orientations can incorporate cognitive and behavioral strategies into their clinical armamentarium without feeling that they must subscribe to a given theory. Techniques can be explained and incorporated by almost any theory. "Technical eclecticism," as Lazarus (1967) has called it, is an approach whereby the clinician borrows techniques from various psychotherapeutic schools. The technically eclectic therapist is willing to employ any technique that is effective.

There has been some research demonstrating the efficacy of cognitive-behavioral interventions for helping cancer patients cope with invasive medical procedures as well as the pain and stress of the disease itself. However, most of the research on cognitive-behavioral interventions has been conducted with other patient populations. Throughout the various chapters we cite the relevant research. However, this is a book for clinicians written by clinicians. Therefore, may of our recommendations are based on our clinical experiences. The methods in this book are those that we have found effective in helping patients cope with cancer.

1

COGNITIVE-BEHAVIORAL THERAPY

We have described our approach as cognitive-behavioral. There are, however, over 10 different cognitive-behavioral approaches (see Dryden & Golden, 1986). Ours might be described as a generic cognitive-behavioral approach, borrowing from the various schools of cognitive-behavioral therapy. We have been most influenced by Ellis' (1962) rational-emotive therapy, Beck's (1976) cognitive therapy, Meichenbaum's (1977) cognitive-behavior modification, the problem-solving approach (D'Zurilla & Goldfried, 1971; Spivack, Platt, & Shure, 1976), Lazarus' (1981) multimodal therapy and Golden's (the senior author of the present book) cognitive-behavioral hypnotherapy (Golden, 1983a; Golden, Dowd, & Friedberg, 1987; Golden & Friedberg, 1986). It is beyond the scope of this book to acquaint the reader with each of these approaches and to discuss their similarities and differences. That has been done elsewhere (see Dryden & Golden, 1986). Instead, we will identify the main concepts and therapeutic strategies from the various cognitive-behavioral approaches relevant in the treatment of cancer patients.

Cognitive-behavioral Assessment

The effectiveness of cognitive-behavioral interventions depends on an adequate assessment. The basics of cognitive-behavioral assessment entail identifying maladaptive thoughts, feelings, behaviors, and physiological reactions as well as the antecedents and reinforcers that maintain them. For the purpose of conceptualizing patients' problems, most cognitive-behavior therapists subscribe to some variation of the S-O-R-C model, where "S" are stimuli or situations in which the patient's problem occurs; "O" are cognitions such as the patient's conscious thoughts (self-statements), irrational beliefs, thinking errors, and underlying assumptions; "R" are responses (emotional, physiological, and behavioral); and "C" are reinforcing consequences such as secondary gains and reactions from other people that undermine the patient's motivation to cope effectively. For example, a patient with terminal cancer sought treatment for depression. Prior to his illness he was a very active, high-functioning individual. But since receiving a diagnosis of cancer he had become depressed, feeling helpless and hopeless. His belief was that a diagnosis of cancer was a "death sentence," to use his own words. Believing he could do nothing, he thought he might as well lie in bed until he died. His family inadvertently reinforced this pattern of thinking, feeling, and acting by encouraging him to be passive and remain bedridden. They catered to him in every way possible, including feeding him and doing all his chores.

The stimulus here was the diagnosis of cancer. The maladaptive cognitions were his beliefs that he was helpless and hopeless which resulted in depression and passivity. His family provided the reinforcement which helped to maintain the pattern. The targets of change were his maladaptive beliefs, his passivity, and the reaction of his family. The interventions included cognitive restructuring (to be discussed shortly) for the maladaptive thinking; problem solving (to be discussed) to reduce helplessness and hopelessness by enabling him to perceive that he did in fact have alternatives other than waiting to die; self-sufficiency and activity therapy for overcoming passivity and helplessness; and counseling to educate the family about how to respond to the patient. The family was instructed to encourage the patient to be active and more self-sufficient. The patient and the family were cooperative and receptive to these interventions. The outcome was that the patient did become more active, pursued most of his prior recreational interests, traveled, returned to work, once again found life meaningful, and was satisfied with his life until his death almost two years later.

The above case is an example of how cognitive-behavioral interventions naturally follow from cognitive-behavioral assessment. The goal is to be as complete as possible in the assessment so as to make the treatment as comprehensive, and therefore as effective, as possible. As Lazarus (1981) has pointed out, the more modalities involved in the treatment, the more effective and enduring will be the therapeutic results. Lazarus has identified seven modalities for therapists to consider: behavior, affect, sensation, imagery, cognition, interpersonal factors, and medication. It may not be appropriate to have treatments for each modality. That depends on the individual case. However, each modality can be assessed to determine what interventions are to become part of the treatment plan. For example, in the above case, although medication was considered, it was not necessary. More will be said about assessment in each of the chapters concerning specific problem areas.

Self-monitoring. Although a large amount of information can be obtained by interviewing the patient, the therapist should not, in most cases, rely entirely on this type of data in the assessment and conceptualization of a patient's problem. Retrospective data can be inaccurate and misleading. Patients are limited in their ability to provide information about their thoughts, feelings, and behaviors when they are not actually experiencing them. Most cognitive-behavior therapists find self-monitoring to be a valuable assessment tool that can be used in conjunction with clinical interviews and self-report questionnaires.

Self-monitoring can be accomplished through different means. Typically, self-monitoring forms (such as those shown in chapter 2 on depression, chapter 3 on stress management, and chapter 4 on pain control) are given to patients to fill out during the week. Patients are taught how to fill them out and explanations are provided as to their importance. The main reason for their use is to gather more accurate information. It is important to explain that the therapist needs this information in order to provide the patient with the most effective treatment possible. The patient, however, may be too ill to cooperate, or there just may not be enough time for self-monitoring. Sometimes situations, such as hospitalization of the patient or impending medical procedures, require rapid intervention from the therapist. Under these conditions flexibility is required. When we have been faced with such situations we have assessed what was needed on the basis of the best available information.

The information sought through self-monitoring depends on the patient's complaint. Usually we are looking for information about the frequency, intensity, duration, and pervasiveness of the patient's complaint. Therefore, for most problems, patients are asked to record the date, time, and situation, as well as their thoughts, feelings, and actions. In addition, they are often asked to rate the intensity of their reactions (pain, anxiety, or depression) and the type and amount of medication they used. Through this type of self-monitoring it is possible to identify the factors that produce or increase the patient's distress, as well as the factors that maintain or reinforce it, such as passivity, drug dependence, or avoidance of responsibilities. Another function of the self-monitoring is to evaluate the effectiveness of the treatment in terms of a reduction in the patient's distress. More will be said about assessment and self-monitoring in each of the chapters on the various problem areas.

Cognitive Restructuring

All cognitive-behavior therapists employ some form of cognitive restructuring. Cognitive-restructuring procedures are techniques for producing cognitive change. Although cognitive restructuring can be accomplished through different means (see Golden & Dryden, 1986), they all are methods for helping individuals to change from maladaptive to more adaptive thinking. The following are the main cognitive-restructuring methods that we use in our work with cancer patients.

The Didactic Method. Through bibliotherapy, or by explanation, misconceptions can be corrected and healthier attitudes can be taught. For example, a therapist may explain to a patient who is feeling guilty over becoming ill that having cancer is not the patient's fault and that he or she did not bring it upon him or herself. Many patients find it helpful to read self-help books that promote healthy attitudes (e.g., Ellis & Harper, 1975).

The Socratic Method. Using Socratic dialogue, the therapist asks thought-provoking questions for the purpose of getting a patient to reevaluate some of his or her self-defeating ideas. For example, the patient who is condemning himself for having cancer might be asked if he would condemn his son or daughter if either of them were ill.

Self-statement Modification. In self-statement modification, maladaptive self-statements are replaced with more adaptive ones. For example, a patient having difficulty coping with chronic pain may be taught to replace catastrophic thoughts that intensify the pain, such as, "I can't stand this pain, it's killing me," with coping self-statements, such as, "It may be distressing but it won't kill me, I can cope with the pain, I can deal with it." Patients are encouraged to participate in the construction of the coping self-statements.

The Two-Column Method. The two-column method is an excellent way of teaching patients how to construct coping self-statements. A page is divided in half. On the left side of the page the patient lists his or her negative self-defeating thoughts. On the right side of the page the patient lists a coping self-statement for each self-defeating thought (for examples, see chapters on depression, stress management, and pain control). The therapist and the patient work together to construct self-statements that the patient will be able to employ in coping with pain, anxiety, or depression. They can be employed by the client whenever he or she is experiencing pain or emotional distress, and can also be part of a broader based stress-management program (to be discussed).

Imagery Rehearsal

There are a number of imagery techniques that can be used in helping cancer patients. Many of them involve having the patient imagine him or herself coping effectively with pain, anxiety, or depression. Combined with relaxation or hypnotic procedures, imagery can be used as part of a stress-management program for reducing pain or for preparing patients for stressful invasive medical procedures, such as chemotherapy, surgery, and bone marrow aspirations. These techniques will be covered in detail throughout the book.

Hypnosis

There are several cognitive-behavioral techniques (described in detail in the chapter on pain control) that are useful in helping patients cope with pain. These methods can be used with or without hypnosis. Golden et al. (1987) have demonstrated how hypnosis and cognitive-behavior therapy are similar and how they can be integrated for the purpose of pain control. Even without employing formal hypnotic procedures, relaxation procedures and imagery have the capacity to reduce at least some pain in most patients.

However, hypnosis has unique value in ameliorating pain. There are several dramatic hypnotic procedures for pain control, such as dissociation, where the patient experiences something that feels like an "out of body" sensation; hypnotic anesthesia, where pain can be eliminated by inducing numbness; and analgesia, involving a dulling of sensation. Some patients are capable of experiencing these phenomena without formal hypnosis, that is, through relaxation and imagery. Nevertheless, although relaxation and hypnosis are similar, many patients believe and expect hypnosis to be powerful in controlling pain. For these individuals, it is more believable that hypnosis will control their pain. In other words, at least in the area of pain control, hypnosis may have more "placebo value" than relaxation alone. Hence, it will be of value for the clinician working with cancer patients to be familiar with some basic hypnotic procedures. We include these in our chapter on pain control but refer the interested reader to Golden et al. (1987) for more information.

Stress Management

Stress- and anxiety-management procedures, such as relaxation techniques, coping self-statements, and mental rehearsal, can be applied to help the cancer patient deal with specific anxieties unrelated to cancer (e.g., job or marital stress) as well as anxieties about having cancer and can be used to help patients cope with invasive medical procedures. Meichenbaum's stress-inoculation training (Meichenbaum, 1977, 1985) and Goldfried's coping-skills approaches to desensitization (Goldfried & Davison, 1976) are particularly effective stress-management procedures. Both techniques are similar. Under relaxed conditions, patients are instructed to imagine themselves coping with stressful events. Through these imagery techniques, patients are given practice in applying relaxation techniques and cognitive-restructuring procedures.

Homework

Homework is an integral part of cognitive-behavior therapy. As mentioned earlier, patients are asked to engage in some type of self-monitoring of thoughts, feelings, and behaviors. Bibliotherapy was also mentioned earlier. Patients are also asked to practice their relaxation techniques and self-hypnosis (if hypnosis is a part of the treatment). Patients are given cassette tapes of the various stress-management and pain-control procedures to listen to at home. Behavioral assignments are given to depressed patients to engage in pleasurable and constructive activity. However, physical activity may or may not be appropriate for patients experiencing pain and those patients in the final stages of their illness. For some patients, physical activity may make them feel worse and intensify pain. Consideration is to be given to the individual needs and physical limitations of the patient prior to prescribing behavioral assignments.

SPECIAL CONSIDERATIONS IN TREATING CANCER PATIENTS

We have found that cancer patients are generally cooperative, highly motivated, and responsive to treatment. Most of them are in treatment through their own volition. They usually follow through on their assignments and usually obtain rapid results. Resistance due to secondary gain tends to be the exception, rather than the rule. Most cancer patients are grateful for whatever help or relief from their suffering we can provide. For these reasons we find our work with them to be very rewarding.

However, there are several issues that may or may not become obstacles to treatment depending on how the clinician handles them. As Cleeland and Tearnan (1986) point out, in overcoming a cancer patient's reluctance to participate in behavioral treatment, it is very important to treat them as medical patients and not as psychotherapy patients. Referral to a psychologist or psychotherapist can lead to misinterpretation. The patient may incorrectly conclude, "My doctor thinks I'm mentally sick," "I'm complaining too much," "I'm not being cooperative," "I'm not trying hard enough," or "The pain is all in my head." The patient may fear that his or her pain medication will be discontinued or reduced.

In the very first session, the clinician can assess what the referral meant to the patient and then disabuse him or her of any misconceptions. We have found it helpful to universalize the patient's reactions and to point out that anyone diagnosed as having cancer would experience a great deal of stress and mental anguish and that their reactions are "normal" and understandable given the traumatic nature of the experience. Patients suffering from pain can be reassured that they will not be forced or be expected to reduce their pain medication as part of their participation in cognitive-behavioral treatment. In actual practice, we find that these patients need all the help they can get in coping with their pain which usually increases as the illness progresses. Therefore, we encourage them to use everything at their disposal, including medication, cognitive-behavioral interventions, and hypnosis.

Many cancer patients seeking relief from pain will find hypnosis to be more acceptable than cognitive-behavioral therapy, not only, as mentioned earlier, because hypnosis may have greater "placebo value" but also because of its association with the treatment of medical problems. Most lay people are aware that hypnosis has a long history of use in the treatment of physical pain and medical problems. Cognitive-behavior therapy does not yet have this association in the public's eyes. However, if the clinician feels uncomfortable about employing hypnosis, he or she can explain that behavioral strategies, such as relaxation procedures, are effective in treating physical pain. In chapter 4 on pain control, we will show how the clinician without formal training in hypnosis may still be able to employ several hypnotic interventions.

Similar issues need to be addressed in treating patients who have developed conditioned aversive reactions as a result of chemotherapy. It has been reported that between 20% and 50% of patients receiving chemotherapy develop anticipatory nausea, and even possibly vomiting, as a result of respondent classical conditioning (Burish & Carey, 1986; Morrow, 1982; Nesse, Carli, Curtis, & Kleinman, 1980; Redd, 1988). These symptoms occur in anticipation of receiving further chemotherapy. They can become attached to what were previously neutral stimuli, such as the doctor's waiting room, the sound of the nurse's voice, or the sight of the treatment room. Feelings of helplessness and shame often can result. Again, we have found universalizing the phenomena to be quite reassuring to the patient. Simply explaining that this is a frequently occurring side effect of chemotherapy, controllable through cognitive-behavioral strategies, reduces the patient's feelings of helplessness and personal failure. In chapter 3, we present a stress-management program that is very effective in helping patients with these conditioned aversive reactions.

The feeling of helplessness is pervasive for cancer patients. Most patients feel that they have no control over their illness, their bodies, and their lives. Feelings of helplessness are exacerbated by the invasive nature of their medical treatments and by their inability to actively participate in their treatment. Addressing these feelings, and explaining how cognitive-behavioral treatment will make them active participants, will help their morale and encourage cooperation. Emphasizing the need for a collaboration between patient and therapist is particularly important when employing hypnosis as part of the treatment. Many people believe and expect that the patient is passive in hypnosis. However, passivity on the part of the patient can interfere with the efficacy of hypnosis. To be maximally effective, the patient needs to practice and apply it. The issue of dealing with the feeling of helplessness will be addressed throughout the book.

Our introduction was not intended to be an all-inclusive discussion of cognitive-behavioral procedures. Likewise, we did not intend to identify each and every issue related to treating cancer patients. Rather, we only wanted to acquaint the reader with the major techniques and some of the key issues. This material and much more will be discussed in greater depth in subsequent chapters.

Chapter 2
Depression

There are many signs of depression. The symptoms can be categorized into four areas:

1. Emotional symptoms, such as a depressed mood or excessive crying.
2. Cognitive symptoms, such as low self-esteem and unrealistic self-criticism. The person sees him or herself as totally responsible for all the problems that are occurring in his or her life. Ellis (1962) and Beck, Rush, Shaw, and Fmery (1979) argue that it is the patient's perceptions, beliefs, and cognitive style that create the depression.
3. Behavioral symptoms, such as lethargy and poor motivation. The patient finds it difficult to engage in activities of daily living.
4. Physical symptoms, such as appetite or sleep disturbance. The patient may eat or sleep either very little or excessively.

Whereas many depressed patients will have a number of these symptoms, some depressions are very subtle. The patient may not feel depressed but may exhibit a few of the behavioral symptoms and the physical symptoms of depression.

BIOCHEMICAL DEPRESSION

Even in individuals who seem to have good reasons for being depressed, a biochemical imbalance may still be a contributing factor. If there are physical symptoms or suicidal ideation, then a formal psychiatric evaluation is indicated to determine whether medication is necessary. Some of the signs of a biochemical imbalance are early-morning awakening, loss of appetite, loss of sex drive, and/or a general malaise. Other symptoms include impaired concentration, a worsening of symptoms in the morning, excessive eating, and a family history of depression.

PSYCHOLOGICAL DEPRESSION

The term "reactive depression" refers to a type of depression occurring in response to a loss, rejection, failure, or disappointment. Many people believe that such losses automatically lead to depression.

Cognitive therapists (Beck, Rush, Shaw & Emery, 1979; Ellis, 1962) view depression as the result of faulty thinking. The individual does not simply become depressed because of a loss or as a result of having cancer. How the individual reacts depends on how that individual perceives and interprets the situation. Ellis and Harper (1975) have made a distinction between sadness and depression. Ellis and Harper (1975) say that sadness is the appropriate response to an event like having cancer or the loss of a loved one. Sadness is adaptive because it motivates one to do something about the situation, such as continuing to enjoy life as much as possible despite having cancer. Depression, on the other hand, is maladaptive because it results in withdrawal and immobility. Cognitive-behavioral strategies have been found to be as effective, or more effective, in treating depression than antidepressant medications (Beck, Hollon, Young, & Bedrosian, 1985; Blackburn, Bishop, Glen, Whalley, & Christie, 1981; Dunn, 1979; Rush, Beck, Kovacs, & Hollon, 1977).

COGNITIVE-BEHAVIORAL CLASSIFICATION OF DEPRESSION

Several patterns of thinking associated with depression can be identified. They can be classified according to whether they involve self-condemnation, hopelessness, or self-pity.

Self-condemnation

Feelings of inadequacy and guilt are two types of depression that are the result of self-condemnation. Some cancer patients feel guilty because they believe they are responsible for having developed cancer. The guilt may stem from a belief that the patient did not take proper care of him or herself. This belief may have some validity, for example, in the case of the cigarette smoker who develops lung cancer. However, there may be little basis in reality for the patient's belief. One therapeutic intervention is to correct a patient's mistaken belief that he or she was responsible. In those cases where the patient's behavior did play a contributing role, such as in cigarette smoking, the cognitive-behavior therapy intervention is to help the patient to be more self-accepting. In cognitive therapy, especially Ellis' (1962) rational-emotive therapy, patients are taught that even if they did do wrong or made a mistake, that does not make them bad or worthless.

Patients are encouraged to accept themselves as fallible human beings who acted with weakness and made mistakes.

Whereas guilt stems from self-condemnation for presumably having done wrong, feelings of inadequacy are based on that belief that one is "worth less" than others. Sometimes a rejection from a significant person in one's life serves as a stimulus for feeling inadequate. For example, one young lady's fiancé terminated their engagement after he learned that she had Hodgkin's disease. She was depressed, believing that she was "stigmatized" and "worthless." Her medical treatments were successful and she was declared by her oncologist to be "cured." Nevertheless, she still felt inadequate. The focus of cognitive-behavioral treatment was to help her stop condemning herself as inadequate and worthless and to get her to begin dating again, which she did.

Feelings of inadequacy can also occur in the absence of rejection from others. Some individuals anticipate others will be rejecting and condemning. It is their own negative feelings about themselves that they project onto others. An example is a woman who avoided sex with her husband after having a mastectomy because she anticipated rejection from him.

In some cases, like the one above, just encouraging communication between the couple and clarifying inaccurate assumptions will remedy the situation. However, in individuals with very low self-esteem, corrective experiences are often not enough. In individuals with long-standing feelings of inadequacy, a lengthier, more intensive cognitive-behavioral treatment is often necessary. In such cases, the therapist addresses the multitude of events about which the patient condemns him or herself. The therapist repeatedly helps the patient to reevaluate these situations, many of which will not be related to having cancer, and encourages the patient to adopt a more accepting attitude.

Hopelessness

Individuals become depressed when they believe they are helpless and hopeless. These beliefs are maladaptive because they depress the individual and become self-fulfilling. The cancer patient who believes that treatment is hopeless will give up. Hope is restored when the individual believes there are alternatives. For example, a woman who required chemotherapy after having a mastectomy started to feel hopeless when the treatment was not 100% effective. The therapist encouraged her to discuss an alternative method of treatment with her oncologist. When she realized that there were alternatives, she began to feel less helpless and hopeless.

Self-pity

Self-pity often comes from magnification (Beck, 1976), or catastrophizing as Ellis (Ellis & Harper, 1975) calls it, about one's problems. Both of these terms relate to exaggeration about one's problems. Self-pity is often manifested by statements such as "why me?" Instead of positive and constructive action, a self-pitying patient will often become lethargic and passive, thus making the situation worse. Many of these patients magnify their illness and assume death is inevitable. Treatment can be directed toward helping the patient realize that he or she can still enjoy life and be productive despite having cancer.

THE DIAGNOSIS AND
ASSESSMENT OF DEPRESSION

The above classification of depression as originating from biochemical factors and psychological factors stemming from self-condemnation, hopelessness, and self-pity is a useful means of identifying and diagnosing different forms of depression. Depending on the diagnosis, treatment can be tailored to the individual patient. Certain interventions are appropriate for depressions involving feelings of hopelessness and helplessness, while others are more appropriate for patients with feelings of inadequacy. These interventions will be discussed later in the chapter. Of course, medication should be considered whenever biochemical signs are present.

Self-report measures such as the Beck Depression Inventory (BDI) (Beck et al., 1979) and the Hopelessness Scale (HS) developed by Beck, Weissman, Lester, and Trexler (1974) can be used to measure depression. The HS has been found to be more accurate for identifying suicidal patients (see Beck, Kovacs, & Weissman, 1975) and seems to be measuring a different type of depression than the BDI. The BDI contains many items about self-condemnation, whereas the HS measures hopelessness and helplessness.

Thus we are able to distinguish different types of depression that are associated with different types of cognitions: self-condemnation which is best measured by the BDI, hopelessness which is best measured by the HS, and self-pity for which, at the present time, there is no self-report measure. The advantage of a cognitive-behavioral diagnosis is that the therapist is then able to employ interventions that are maximally effective with that particular type of depression. For example, we have often seen our supervisees attempting to help patients stop self-deprecating when their depression was really the result of feeling hopeless and helpless. Therapists, especially novice cognitive-behavior therapists, often incorrectly conclude that if a patient is depressed they must be engaging in self-deprecation. Effective cognitive restructuring requires targeting the correct maladaptive cognitions.

Self-monitoring

Self-monitoring involves the identification and recording of the situations and maladaptive cognitions that lead to disturbing feelings and self-defeating behaviors. In depression, the negative appraisals of oneself, the future, and the world are often in the forefront of consciousness. We have categorized them as either involving self-condemnation, helplessness and hopelessness, or self-pity. With very little training and practice, most depressed patients can be taught to observe their conscious cognitions which are in the form of an "internal dialogue" or what Beck et al. (1979) calls "automatic thoughts."

Patients are instructed whenever they feel depressed to identify and write down, either in a log or on self-monitoring sheets, their automatic thoughts. Table 2.1 is a self-monitoring form that can be used to monitor maladaptive thoughts and feelings. A scale, rating Subjective Units of Discomfort (SUDS levels), can be used to rate how depressed, anxious, or angry an individual feels. The patient rates on a scale from 0 to 100% how depressed they feel at a given moment. The rational response column will be used for cognitive restructuring.

Evocative Imagery

Evocative imagery can help patients to reexperience what they actually thought and felt in the real-life situation. In addition, this method may have an advantage over self-monitoring, at least in the initial stages of therapy, in that a patient may feel more secure in examining his or her disturbing thoughts and feelings in the presence of a supportive therapist.

In employing evocative imagery, the patient is instructed to imagine a situation in which he or she recently felt depressed. The patient is encouraged to feel whatever he or she felt in the real-life situation, notice whatever thoughts and feelings come to mind, and report them to the therapist as they are experienced.

An example of the use of evocative imagery occurred when John was asked about his depression. He reported that he was in his physician's office, being told by the physician that more chemotherapy was needed. Initially, John could not identify any thoughts and could only say he felt depressed. However, when John was asked to imagine the situation, he was then able to connect having felt depressed with thoughts that he was

Table 2.1. Self-Monitoring Form
Situation: Patient Being Told More Chemotherapy Is Needed

Situation	Feelings Rate degree of feelings 1–100%	Automatic Thought(s)	Rational Response	Outcome Rerate Feelings
Told by doctor that I must have more chemotherapy than expected.	Depression 85%	1. The chemotherapy is not working. (hopelessness)	1. Some people require more chemotherapy than others and my body is responding positively.	Sad 30%
		2. The doctor is lying to me about the severity of my condition.	2. The doctor is telling me what he knows. He is not able to accurately predict treatment outcome.	
		3. Poor me. Everything happens to me.	3. That's self-pity and it's not true. I've had disappoint-ments but I do have positive things going for me, such as my job and my family.	

hopeless and would soon die. The therapist suggested that he might be interpreting the situation incorrectly and recommended that the patient check out his beliefs with the physician. See the next section and Table 2.1 for examples of how the therapist used cognitive restructuring, which is the next step after the patient's maladaptive thoughts and feelings are elicited through self-monitoring or evocative imagery.

COGNITIVE RESTRUCTURING

One of the purposes of the self-monitoring forms is to help patients to identify maladaptive attitudes, thoughts, and beliefs. Although the identification of these maladaptive cognitions can have therapeutic effects, usually such insight is insufficient for reducing depression. Usually, some type of cognitive restructuring is needed. Most cognitive-restructuring procedures involve some method of helping patients to replace self-defeating patterns of thinking with more constructive ways of thinking. There are several cognitive-restructuring procedures applicable to the treatment of depression.

Self-statement Modification

Self-statement modification can be accomplished by using the same self-monitoring form that was described earlier in the chapter for identifying automatic thoughts. Patients are first instructed to monitor situations in which they feel depressed, rate the intensity of depression felt in the situation, and record their automatic thoughts.

After patients are able to successfully monitor and record the necessary information about precipitating events and thoughts that lead to depression, they can be taught how to construct rational coping self-statements. Patients are instructed to question and reevaluate their automatic thoughts and to arrive at a rational response which can be used to neutralize the automatic thoughts. They write down these rational self-statements in the rational response column and are instructed to employ them whenever they experience the corresponding automatic thoughts. If the patient experiences automatic thoughts that are different from those on the form, the patient can then fill out a new form and generate additional rational self-statements. In this manner, the patient not only learns to modify specific self-statements but also learns a method that can be used to combat other automatic thoughts.

See Table 2.1 for an example of a self-monitoring form for self-statement modification. John, the patient whose automatic thoughts and rational responses are presented in Table 2.1, was depressed because he was informed by his physician that he needed more chemotherapy than was originally planned. John rated his depression at a SUDS level of 85%. In this case, the patient was able to identify three automatic thoughts:

1. "The chemotherapy is not working and I'm hopeless."
2. "My doctor is lying to me about the severity of my condition."
3. "Poor me, everything happens to me."

In the rational response column, the patient is asked to record those rational statements that he could use to dispute the irrational automatic thoughts, thus reducing his feeling of depression. With the help of the therapist, John was able to arrive at the following rational statements:

1. "Some people require more chemotherapy than others and my body is responding positively."
2. "The doctor is telling me what he knows. He isn't able to accurately predict treatment results."
3. "That's self-pity and it's not true. I've had disappointments, but I do have positive things going for me, such as my career and my family."

The final column requires the patient to report the outcome from the cognitive restructuring. In this case, depression became sadness with a

SUDS level of 30%. Rerating the intensity of the feeling is important so that patients can see that feelings do not have all-or-none existences. This provides patients with a realistic model of change. Patients usually do not suddenly give up irrational beliefs and eliminate automatic thoughts as a result of being given a rational response or arriving at one on their own. Rather, change occurs in small steps.

Two-column Method

Many patients prefer the two-column method over the more elaborate self-monitoring form because it is less complicated. The patient is instructed to divide a page in half (see Table 2.2).

At the top of the page, the patient writes a brief description of the situation. On the left side of the page the patient lists his or her automatic thoughts and/or irrational beliefs that caused the depression. The patient reevaluates each maladaptive thought and in the other column lists rational responses to each thought. The idea is to construct rational self-statements that will counteract the depressive effect of the maladaptive thoughts. For the purpose of providing a comparison between the self-monitoring form and the two-column method, John's automatic thoughts and rational responses from Table 2.1 are rearranged in Table 2.2.

Imagery Rehearsal

Imagery can be used to prepare patients for coping with situations in which they typically become depressed. The therapist helps the patient anticipate events that could be a problem. Through methods such as those just previously discussed, a list of rational coping self-statements are constructed which are then used by the patient during the imagery. This

Table 2.2. Sample Two-Column Method
Situation: Being Told By Doctor That More Chemotherapy Is Needed

Automatic Thoughts	Rational Statements
1. The chemotherapy is not working (hopelessness).	1. Some people require more chemotherapy than others and my response to treatment is still positive.
2. The doctor is lying to me about the severity of my condition.	2. The doctor is telling me what he knows. He is not able to accurately predict treatment outcome.
3. Poor me. Everything happens to me.	3. That's self-pity and it's not true. I've had disappointments but I do have positive things going for me, such as my job and my family.

imagery technique provides the patient with an opportunity to mentally rehearse how to think and act in the situation, and increases the likelihood that he or she will successfully cope with it. Patients seem to undergo more cognitive change when imagery rehearsal is employed than when self-statement modification is used alone. Meichenbaum (1977) has emphasized the importance of providing patients with some type of opportunity to rehearse coping strategies prior to confronting stressful situations.

As an illustration of imagery rehearsal, John, the man whose automatic thoughts and rational self-statements were described in Table 2.1 and Table 2.2, will once again be used as an example. As you may recall, John was depressed over being told by his physician that he needed more chemotherapy. Especially difficult for him was the thought that he was different than other cancer patients who probably needed less treatment.

Through the use of imagery, John anticipated how he could cope with self-pity and feelings of hopelessness. During the imagery, he mentally rehearsed how he wanted to think, feel, and act when actually involved in the chemotherapy process. John practiced employing the rational coping self-statements in Table 2.1 and Table 2.2, and imagined himself feeling sad instead of depressed.

John was instructed to practice using the rational coping self-statements and the imagery-rehearsal techniques at least once a day, on his own, for homework. This technique enabled him to get over feeling depressed and allowed him to engage in chemotherapy treatment with a much more positive attitude.

Although many patients respond to cognitive-restructuring techniques rapidly, others do not. It often takes patients continuous effort, over a period of time, before they start to feel better.

The Didactic Method

Another method that can be employed in getting patients to rationally reevaluate their faulty thinking is the didactic method. The therapist corrects misperceptions, faulty assumptions, and irrational beliefs, then suggests more rational ways of viewing the situation.

A didactic approach was taken with a female patient who was depressed about receiving a diagnosis of breast cancer. The following is the dialogue that occurred:

Patient: I feel that nothing is important anymore.
Therapist: Your illness is serious, but you have a lot going for you. You told me you have a great family, a good job, and great friends.
Patient: Well, that's true, but none of it matters now that I'm going to die.
Therapist: You don't know you're going to die. You haven't been told that by your doctor.

Patient: Why do these things always happen to me? I'm doomed.
Therapist: It's not true that only negative things happen to you, and you're not doomed. Treatment for breast cancer is very effective today.
Patient: I know you're right. I guess I'm really scared about the future.
Therapist: That's understandable.

The Socratic Method

Another way of helping patients question and reevaluate their faulty thinking is by using the Socratic method. The Socratic method entails eliciting rational responses from patients as a result of getting them to question their thinking. This technique gets the patient to reevaluate incorrect assumptions, misperceptions, and irrational beliefs. The therapist would not rush in so readily to correct the patient's faulty thinking as he or she might if employing a didactic approach. Instead, the therapist tries to help the patient arrive at the rational responses.

A Socratic approach to the previous dialogue could have gone like this:

Patient: I feel that nothing is important anymore.
Therapist: Your illness is serious, but don't you have family, friends, and a good job?
Patient: Well, that's true, but none of it matters now that I'm going to die.
Therapist: What makes you think you are going to die? What did your doctor say?
Patient: He said success rates were high and that I really stand a good chance of not having cancer in the future.
Therapist: When you think about it that way, how do you feel?
Patient: If I look at it that way, I do feel less depressed. I guess I'm scared about the future.
Therapist: That's understandable.

Whereas some clients respond better to a Socratic approach, others prefer more direction. Trial and error is sometimes required before the therapist is able to assess which style is more appropriate with a given patient. Furthermore, there are times when, even with the same patient, the therapist may find it most effective to switch styles. For example, if being Socratic does not elicit the right answer, it makes sense for the therapist to provide it. Alternatively, at the beginning of therapy, the therapist often has to be more didactic and provide direction. As therapy progresses, the patient is more capable of assuming greater responsibility, so the therapist can become more Socratic.

BEHAVIORAL TECHNIQUES

Activity Therapy

A strategy used in cognitive-behavior therapy to relieve depression is to get patients to do things that are pleasurable and constructive (Beck et al., 1979). There are a number of activities that patients can engage in that help reduce depression. We have found that, if the patient is able, going back to work is one of the most beneficial activities. Apparently, working at one's profession restores and maintains positive feelings. Engaging in constructive activity is a way that patients can reduce feelings of inadequacy and helplessness. In addition, when one returns to the work place there is often a lessening of tension in the home as the family does not feel the burden of being totally responsible for the patient.

If the patient is capable of exercise, this will also help restore positive feelings. This is most dramatic in those patients who were quite active before the disease. Active patients are less likely to passively feel sorry for themselves and "wait to die."

The effectiveness of activity was demonstrated with a female patient depressed about having breast cancer which had metastasized. With the support of her therapist, she decided to seek employment within the scope of her physical capabilities. Though the job was not demanding or well-paid, she immediately felt less depressed once she began work.

Pleasurable activity also has the capacity to reduce depression. It has been hypothesized that depression stems from a lack of positive experiences and therefore a lack of reinforcers in the environment (Ferster, 1973; Lewinsohn, 1974).

Some caution is needed when recommending activity therapy to cancer patients. The therapist should be aware of the patient's physical limitations by speaking with his or her physician. This will prevent suggesting an activity that the patient will be unable to perform or one that may cause pain or injury. More will be said about this in the chapter on pain control.

Time Projection

Some patients are unable to respond to directives to be more active. Some are too depressed. Lazarus' (1968) time-projection technique can be used to elevate the mood and energy level of the very depressed patient enough so that he or she can become more active. In addition, it may instill hope. This can occur because the patient visualizes him or herself in the future.

The patient is asked to imagine him or herself engaging in pleasurable and constructive activity in the near future, such as the next week, next month, or possibly several months away. The images can involve pleasurable experiences and the attainment of goals.

The material for the time-projection procedure is taken from the patient's own experiences. A hypnotic procedure may be used prior to the time projection although it is not necessary. If hypnosis is to be used, energizing suggestions as opposed to suggestions of relaxation seem more effective (see Golden et al., 1987, for details). Because relaxation produces a low-arousal state, and depression is already a low-arousal state, relaxation procedures can cause more depression. Therefore, the patient imagines him or herself being active and energized during the time-projection procedure. The therapist describes several images. For example:

"Close your eyes and imagine that you are swimming. You are by the lake feeling a cool refreshing breeze against your body, breathing fresh country air. Now you are walking into the lake and feeling the cool refreshing water. You dive in and feel the cool fresh water, making your body come alive. Now imagine that you are at home. It's sometime this week and you are listening to your favorite music. You are really enjoying the music and you remember some positive experiences associated with this song. Now imagine sometime later the same week. You pick up a cookbook and start to plan a dinner party for some close friends, getting more pleasure and enjoyment out of the activity."

Goal Setting

Patients are encouraged to establish goals and start working toward them. Hope is engendered by the setting and pursuit of goals. Goal setting is similar to activity therapy, such as when the patient's goal is to return to work or start an exercise program. In addition, goal setting can involve desires that patients always wanted to fulfill but never did, such as writing a book, traveling, or volunteering at a community agency. Some cancer patients are reluctant about establishing goals for the future because they feel that they will not be around to enjoy the experience. If this is the case, the therapist can take the position that quality of life is important, regardless of how long one may live. For example, a woman patient always wanted to go to Europe and thought the idea was hopeless now that she had cancer. With the encouragement of the therapist and her husband, she planned the European trip. This greatly reduced feelings of hopelessness. She completed the trip prior to her death 9 months later. Her husband reported that the two of them were very grateful to have had that last positive experience together.

Working With Family

It is important to counsel family members to not infantilize the cancer patient, but rather to encourage him or her to continue to function. This type of activity therapy and family counseling is effective in reducing feelings of hopelessness and helplessness.

An example of this approach was described in the introduction. Prior to his illness, a patient with terminal cancer was a very active, high-functioning individual. However, he became depressed after the diagnosis, believing he could do nothing but stay at home and wait to die. His family inadvertently reinforced this belief by encouraging him to remain passive and bedridden. The family was counseled about how to encourage appropriate activity. The patient became more active, self-sufficient, returned to work, and once again found life meaningful until his death almost 2 years later. More will be said about treating the family in the chapter on family counseling.

DEPRESSION AND IMPLICATIONS FOR CANCER

The Cancer-prone Personality

During the past several years, researchers have attempted to establish a link between psychological factors and incidence of cancer. Several researchers have found that cancer-prone individuals are less assertive, suppress negative emotions, and are more willing to accept outside authority (Kneier & Temoshok, 1984; Temoshok, Heller, Sagebiel, Blois, Sweet, DiClemente, & Gold, 1985). Other researchers report that cancer-prone individuals are often incapable of dealing with anger and hostility, and often feel hopeless or lose their "reason for being" in response to traumatic life events, such as the loss of a loved one (Grossarth-Maticek, Bastiaans, & Kanazir, 1985; Grossarth-Maticek, Schmidt, Vetter, & Arndt, 1984; Grossarth-Maticek, Siegrest, & Vetter, 1982; LeShan, 1977). The position taken by these researchers is that certain traits associated with depression and depressive reactions in response to traumatic losses predispose individuals to developing cancer.

Scheng and Blohmke (1988) using interview techniques found that certain traumas, such as the death of one's mother before age 16, divorce, or separation, seemed to be associated with the development of cancer. The authors acknowledge that the results are inconclusive because they could not be certain if prior events actually caused cancer. Shekelle, Raynor, and Ostfeld (1981) in a 17-year follow-up and Persky, Kempthorne-Rawson, and Shekelle (1987) in a 20-year follow-up of 2,020 men found a two-fold increase in the risk of death from cancer associated with scores on the depression scale of the Minnesota Multiphasic Personality Inventory. However, these results were not duplicated in a 10-year follow-up study by Zonderman, Costa, and McCrae (1989). Using the Center for Epidemiologic Studies Depression Scale and the depression subscale from the General Well-being Schedule, Zonderman et al. (1989) failed to find a significant correlation between depression and cancer morbidity or mortality. In addition, the data were analyzed for those people age 55 and older in a 15-year follow-up with similar results.

It appears that although some researchers have found an association between traumatic life events, depression, and cancer, it has not been established that depression or traumatic losses cause cancer.

Programs That Prolong Life

A related issue is whether or not relieving depression in cancer patients will prolong life or contribute to remissions. According to LeShan (1977), psychotherapy can help patients to fight their cancer. In LeShan's "crisis therapy," he focuses on helping patients alter their lifestyle so they will be more assertive, independent, and regain meaning in life. He reports that patients become more capable of fighting cancer when they make these changes. In addition, his treatment focuses on patients' strengths rather than their weaknesses. By identifying strengths and encouraging a positive outlook, patients are provided with hope. The identified strengths can also be used for future activities and goal setting. LeShan asserts that cancer patients are too often told what they can not accomplish. According to LeShan, the role of the therapist is to help cancer patients to believe in themselves, which in turn promotes healthy risk-taking behavior.

Siegel (1986) believes strongly in the power of the patient to control his or her disease. He suggests that "instead of turning fighters into victims, we should be turning victims into fighters." In his treatment approach, he helps patients fight their cancer by being more positive, assertive, and feeling better about themselves. In addition, he uses techniques similar to those developed by Simonton, Simonton, and Creighton (1978). He believes that patients should learn how to open up emotionally and stop hiding their feelings, as he reports so many cancer patients are prone to do. Although he has little scientific evidence to confirm his hypotheses, he can point to many cases where patients have made remarkable psychological changes and survived despite the odds against their doing so.

Simonton et al. (1978) have developed an approach that they claim both prolongs and improves the quality of life for cancer patients. Their procedure involves the use of healing imagery. Patients are taught relaxation skills and visualization. They are encouraged to create their own healing images. This imagery could be anatomically correct, like one of our patients who used images of the chemotherapy breaking down cancer cells. Images can also be totally based on fantasy. For example, some patients imagine piranha-like cells, that resemble little video game "Pac Men," consuming the cancer cells in the affected part of the body. The image could also be symbolic. Some patients use their relaxation image to symbolize healing. For example, one patient's image was of a special place on the coast of Maine, where there are tidal pools. Tidal pools were symbolic of a healing force for him. Other aspects of the Simonton program include learning to be more assertive, setting goals, learning to manage pain, embarking on an exercise program, and learning how to utilize one's family as a support system.

The rationale behind the program seems to be that patients have greater control over their lives than they might otherwise believe they had. Simonton et al. (1978) advise patients to continue in traditional medical care, using the Simonton program as a supplement.

Cousins (1989) reports in his book of a study by Fawzy, Fahey, Morton, and Cousins undertaken at the University of California at Los Angeles, in which it was found that psychotherapy with cancer patients had rather dramatic effects on depression, quality of life, and immune-cell changes. The therapy included various relaxation techniques as well as positive coping strategies, such as problem-solving techniques, learning how to fight the illness (i.e., "don't deny the diagnosis, just defy the verdict that is supposed to accompany it"), and learning how to laugh. The patients receiving this treatment had significantly lower tension-anxiety and depression scores than no therapy controls. Furthermore, quality of life was assessed as higher in the experimental group and there was a significant difference in immune-cell activity for the experimental group versus the controls.

Changes in the immune system, as a result of relaxation training, have also been reported by Gruber, Hall, Hersh, and Dubois (1988). Cancer patients were taught relaxation and were instructed to imagine forces in their immune system fighting the cancer cells. The researchers report that this treatment increased antibodies, interluken-2 cells, stimulated lymphocytes, enhanced natural killer (NK) cell activity, and augmented the effectiveness of cytotoxic T cells.

Spiegel, Bloom, Kraemer, and Gottheil (1989) report that supportive group therapy (which included self-hypnosis for pain control, assertiveness training, and encouragement to express grief and other feelings) was effective in prolonging life in patients with metastatic breast cancer. The researchers also note that the group-therapy patients developed strong relationships with one another which may have been an important factor. The difference in survival rate for the experimental group versus a control group, which only received medical treatment, was statistically significant.

The group-therapy patients survived an average of 36.6 months, whereas the patients in the control group survived an average of 18.9 months.

Commonalities of Programs That Prolong Life

There are a number of similarities between the various programs reported to prolong life or strengthen the immune system. Some type of assertiveness training is usually part of the treatment. Most of them address the patient's grief and depression in some manner. In addition, most of the programs include stress-management procedures similar to those that will be described in the next chapter. Furthermore, these programs also directly or indirectly provide social support and encourage the development of new relationships. Spiegel et al. (1989) and Cousins (1989) have suggested that forming relationships with other cancer patients may be an important factor in helping patients cope with cancer and may help prolong life.

Hazards of Programs for Prolonging Life

One of the problems facing the therapist working with cancer patients is knowing how to raise hope without instilling false hope. On the one hand, it is important to encourage positive thinking, although one also does not want to build false expectations. Whether or not techniques such as the Simonton method truly improve a patient's chances of overcoming cancer, it apparently helps many cancer patients to feel more hopeful and more in control of their lives. Cousins (1989) and Siegel (1986) assert that when people feel more hopeful and have more positive attitudes they are better fighters. Most oncologists that we have worked with are highly in favor of any method that will encourage positive thinking in their patients.

On the other hand, some of the literature on psychological factors in cancer has contributed to some patients feeling guilty about having cancer. For example, Simonton's work in treating cancer patients through imagery and meditation is sometimes misinterpreted by patients to mean, "If I can use meditation procedures to cope with cancer or cure cancer, then I must have caused the cancer or failed to cure myself of it." Cassileth, Lusk, Miller, Brown, and Miller (1985), who found no relationship between psychological factors and length of survival or remission, feel that methods like those used by Simonton can lead to guilt on the part of cancer patients if they fail to alter the course of their disease. This guilt can be quite devastating, leading to severe depression. The therapist can make a distinction between using self-control procedures for coping with cancer and using them to cure cancer. It is important to help patients to realize that it is a theory and not an established fact that cancer is either caused by depression or that cancer can be cured by psychological methods.

What Programs for Prolonging Life Have to Offer Cognitive-Behavior Therapy

Cognitive-behavioral treatment programs can and do incorporate some of the methods and concepts from these programs. Cognitive-behavioral treatment for depression, including feelings of helplessness and hopelessness, were described earlier in the chapter. Teaching patients how to set goals is another technique that is used in cognitive-behavior therapy. Goal-setting is an important component of any plan for changing behavior and is useful for instilling hope for the future.

Most cancer patients would also benefit from assertiveness training. Many patients have trouble communicating important feelings to their physicians, members of their family, associates in their work place as well as others. It is beyond the scope of this book to teach assertiveness training. Those readers unfamiliar with the literature can consult Fensterheim and Baer (1975) and Lange and Jakubowski (1976) for detailed descriptions of assertiveness training.

Cognitive-behavior therapy techniques may help prolong life even when they are not intentionally being used for that purpose. Programs that have included healing imagery have also included cognitive-behavioral techniques, such as relaxation and assertiveness training. However, it may not be necessary to use healing imagery at all. Cousins (1989) reports that relaxation and other coping strategies were found to be effective in producing changes in the immune system and quality of life in cancer patients. Spiegel et al. (1989) report that the combination of self-hypnosis for pain relief and supportive group therapy was effective in prolonging life. Neither of these programs included healing imagery. Furthermore, in the Spiegel et al. (1989) study, the patients were not led to believe that the treatment would prolong life. Perhaps stress management, assertiveness training, and other cognitive-behavioral interventions may be all that is needed to affect the immune system and prolong life.

SUMMARY

This chapter has focused on the definition and diagnosis of depression. Specific assessment tools were discussed along with cognitive-behavioral treatment procedures. Finally, alternative treatments were outlined and the controversial issues over their validity as scientific theories and their application as clinical tools was discussed.

Chapter 3

Stress Management

Stress is the body's response to demands put upon it. Stress can result from physical or psychological causes. Pain and illnesses such as cancer are examples of physical stressors. In addition, medical treatments for cancer, such as surgery, chemotherapy, and radiation therapy, as well as invasive diagnostic procedures, such as bone marrow aspirations, are experienced by many patients as even more stressful than the disease itself. For example, it has been reported that 20% to 50% of cancer patients develop anticipatory anxiety, nausea, and vomiting from chemotherapy (Burish & Carey, 1986; Morrow, 1982; Nesse, Carli, Curtis, & Kleinman, 1980). Cognitive-behavioral interventions, such as relaxation techniques, cognitive restructuring, and desensitization, can be used to help cancer patients cope with their disease-related and treatment-related stress.

Cognitive processes play a significant role in stress. Stress is typically experienced when the individual perceives him or herself as threatened or in danger. Patients who are more successful in coping with cancer tend to be more positive in their thinking and are willing to take an active role in their medical treatment; whereas, those who have difficulty coping tend to view their situation as hopeless and therefore do not fight or take an active role in treatment (Cousins, 1989; Le Shan, 1977; Siegel, 1986).

BASIC STRESS-MANAGEMENT PROGRAM

The basic components of a stress-management program include the use of relaxation procedures, cognitive methods, and imagery to reduce tension and anxiety. Imagery is particularly useful because it provides

27

patients with the opportunity to prepare themselves for stressful situations.

Several steps occur before patients are taught stress-management skills. Whenever possible, the therapist first conducts a thorough assessment. Patients are taught about stress and are instructed to monitor their stress reactions whenever they occur.

DIAGNOSIS AND ASSESSMENT OF STRESS AND ANXIETY-RELATED SYMPTOMS

An important part of assessment is the determination of how the patient manifests stress. The physical manifestations of stress can be visceral or muscular. A common set of visceral symptoms from stress include increases in heart rate, respiration, blood pressure, sweating, and vasoconstriction of peripheral blood vessels. Muscle tension is another manifestation of stress.

Prior to stress-management training, the therapist conducts as complete an assessment as possible of the stress-related problems being presented by the patient. There are situations, such as a patient needing immediate preparation for an impending medical procedure or a patient needing immediate pain relief, where the assessment must by necessity be brief and therefore incomplete. However, under ideal conditions assessment continues for several sessions, long enough for the therapist to interview the patient and have the patient monitor his or her stress reactions during the week. Although the first session, and possibly the second, is devoted mainly to assessment, the assessment process continues throughout treatment.

The goals of the first session are to begin the assessment process, begin to educate the patient about stress and cognitive-behavioral treatment, and to establish rapport. Cancer patients do not like to be thought of as having psychological problems. In order to establish rapport it is important, whenever possible, to treat the cancer patient's complaints as natural consequences to having cancer. A good starting point is to discuss the patient's medical problems and their medical treatments. Then the therapist can discuss any side effects and stress reactions they have as a result of their chemotherapy or radiation treatment. It is reassuring for the patient to learn that stress reactions are typically experienced as a result of medical treatments for cancer. A stress symptom checklist such as the one in Table 3.1 can be used to help clients identify their particular stress reactions. After identifying a patient's stress-related symptoms, the next step is to identify the specific stressors that elicit these reactions in the patient.

Table 3.1. Stress Symptom Checklist

Below is a list of stress-related symptoms and conditions. If
you are experiencing some of the symptoms below, it may
be an indication that you are having difficulty coping with
your illness. Check the symptoms below which you have
been experiencing recently.

_____ Muscle aches (neck, shoulders, back, legs)
_____ Extreme changes in appetite
_____ Insomnia, nightmares
_____ Increased sweating
_____ Nausea, stomach pain, indigestion
_____ Grinding teeth
_____ Headaches, dizziness
_____ Constipation or diarrhea
_____ Loss of sex drive
_____ High blood pressure, face flushing
_____ Dry mouth or throat
_____ Irritability or bad temper
_____ Lethargy or inability to work
_____ Cold, clammy, or clenched hands
_____ Depression or moodiness
_____ Fear, panic, or anxiety
_____ Fatigue, excessive sleeping
_____ Restlessness
_____ Hyperventilation, shortness of breath
_____ Increased number of minor accidents
_____ Racing thoughts, inability to concentrate
_____ Increased consumption of alcohol or tranquilizers
_____ Increased memory lapses
_____ Increased frequency of mistakes
_____ Changes in habitual behavior
_____ Inability to enjoy work or play
_____ Feelings of hopelessness, uselessness, despair
_____ Thinking constantly about things you cannot
        change
_____ Heart symptoms: acute anxiety attack
_____ Tics, muscle twitches, muscle tension

Self-monitoring

A great deal of information can be obtained through clinical interviews.
However, patients' retrospective reports may be inaccurate and are best
treated as hypotheses to be confirmed or disconfirmed as a result of obtaining more data. A more accurate method of obtaining information about a
patient's maladaptive thoughts, feelings, and actions is to have the patient
log them when they are experienced. We have found that patients are more
likely to comply with requests to self-monitor if the form is a simple one
such as the stress diary in Table 3.2. This form enables patients to record
the situations, thoughts, and feelings that elicit stress reactions.

In addition to providing information for assessment, self-monitoring

Table 3.2. Stress Diary

Day	Time	Situation	Stress Level (0–10)	Thoughts	Feelings	Behavior

serves several other purposes. It sets the stage for the collaborative role that the patient takes in cognitive-behavior therapy. Self-monitoring helps patients to understand the interrelationship between thoughts, feelings, and environmental events. It helps the therapist demonstrate the role that thoughts have in feelings and makes the patient aware of the stimuli serving as "triggers" for maladaptive responses.

Treatment-related Stress

As mentioned at the beginning of the chapter, many patients find chemotherapy very stressful and experience an aversive reaction consisting of nausea and vomiting. These symptoms can become attached to previously neutral situations through what seems to be the result of classical conditioning (Carey & Burish, 1988). For example, one patient became anxious, nauseous, and even sometimes vomited when she saw the nightgown that she wore during chemotherapy or when the nurse called her to make an appointment for another chemotherapy treatment. Another patient became nauseous and anxious at his work place. When he was lying down receiving his chemotherapy, he would look up at the ceiling and see the exact ceiling tiles that were on the ceiling at his work place. Whenever he would look up at the ceiling at work he would experience the same reaction that he had from his chemotherapy treatment. Just the sight of the tiles evoked nausea and anxiety. Desensitization (to be described later) is effective in controlling these reactions. Patients are taught to employ relaxation procedures and coping self-statements to control their reactions to chemotherapy. It is preferable to begin cognitive-behavioral treatment prior to a patient's first chemotherapy treatment because the conditioned aversive reaction can be prevented and treatment can be brief — sometimes only two or three sessions of relaxation training. The aversive reaction to chemotherapy is more difficult to control once it becomes attached to previously neutral stimuli. Nevertheless, even when a conditioned aversive reaction develops, desensitization can be quite effective in its elimination.

Cancer-related Stress

In addition to the stress evoked by the medical treatments, there are stressors related to having cancer. For example, a patient came to see one of the authors after going through radiation for throat cancer. She was a very successful executive in a medium-sized company. She felt self-conscious because her speech was impaired. She was anxious about going to work, feeling that she was not the asset she was before the illness. Part of treatment involved helping her to realize through cognitive restructuring (to be described later) that she was indeed an asset at her job. After returning to work, she recognized that her fears were groundless and that both clients and coworkers accepted her readily. Other stressors to be aware of relate to one's body image after cancer surgery. Women are subject to fears about rejection after undergoing breast surgery. Therapy can help patients overcome fears of rejection and other sexual anxieties. Often the husband is reluctant to pursue his wife only because he senses that she is anxious about sex. Ironically, it is often the case that the wife is afraid because she incorrectly believes that he does not want her. In situations such as these, clarifying incorrect assumptions, which is part of cognitive restructuring, can be very effective in reducing a patient's anxiety about sex.

Another source of stress is the patient's fear of dying. A great deal of sensitivity is required in dealing with anxieties about death. Some patients engage in "constructive" denial. They use positive thinking to combat their fears. Not all denial should be confronted. Often cancer patients use denial constructively to cope with their illness. There are several therapeutic interventions involving the use of positive thinking (to be discussed later) that facilitate "constructive denial." On the other hand, it is very important for the therapist to be able to deal with the subject of death when a patient has a need to talk about it.

Stressors Unrelated to Cancer

Patients may have additional sources of stress that existed prior to their having cancer or may exist independent of the disease. For example, a patient may have had marital or work-related problems before becoming ill. The same techniques can be applied to any type of stress, regardless of its origin.

SKILLS-TRAINING PHASE OF STRESS MANAGEMENT

In stress management, patients are taught specific skills, such as relaxation techniques and cognitive-restructuring procedures that they learn to use as coping tools.

Relaxation Training

Stress has cognitive components (worry or fear) and is experienced viscerally (for example, rapid heart rate, increased sweating, and rapid breathing) and is manifested through the musculature as tension. Physiological components of anxiety are most easily controlled by relaxation procedures. In addition, success in experiencing relaxation can reduce feelings of helplessness and increase a patient's receptivity to other therapeutic interventions (Burish & Lyles, 1979; Cotanch, 1983; Dahlquist, Gil, Armstrong, Ginsberg, & Jones, 1985).

Relaxation procedures that are effective in reducing tension include Jacobson's (1938) progressive relaxation and Goldfried & Davison's (1976) "letting go" relaxation. Breathing techniques are most effective in controlling visceral reactions. Imagery of peaceful scenes and the "mantra" technique (use of a pleasant word such as "calm") are most effective in producing mental relaxation.

There is, of course, some interaction between cognitive, visceral, and muscular systems. Most significant is the visceral relaxation response which Benson (1975) has demonstrated can be produced through mental relaxation techniques. The clinician may either select the relaxation procedures that will be most effective given the specific stress symptoms of the patient or take a "shotgun" approach and use a relaxation procedure that includes progressive muscle relaxation, diaphragmatic breathing, and mental relaxation (pleasant imagery and/or a mantra).

Preparation of the Patient for Relaxation. The preparation of the patient and the physical setting are important considerations. The room should be quiet and lights in the room should be dim. The use of a reclining chair or

comfortable couch is helpful. In addition, it is important to make certain
that the patient is comfortable with the procedure and that rapport between therapist and patient is well established.

We have found the following guidelines helpful in preparing patients
for relaxation training (modified from Goldfried & Davison, 1976).

1. The patient is told he or she is about to learn a new skill much like
    driving a car or riding a bicycle. Learning will be gradual and, like any
    skill, practice is necessary.
2. The therapist informs the patient that different sensations, such as
    tingling and drowsiness, may occur that are all related to the relaxation
    process and not to be afraid of them.
3. The therapist reassures the patient about any fears he or she may have
    regarding relaxation. For example, some patients feel that if they relax,
    they will be unable to control themselves. Reassuring the patient that
    he or she will remain in control even in a deeply relaxed state is often
    sufficient in alleviating this anxiety. Another approach is to perform
    a modified or shortened relaxation exercise. The patient can also be
    reassured that at anytime during the procedure he or she can stop the
    exercise.
4. Eliminate performance demands. The patient can be reassured that
    relaxation skills take time to develop.
5. The patient is told that, during relaxation, stray thoughts may enter
    one's mind. When this occurs, all one has to do is refocus one's atten-
    tion onto the relaxation procedure.
6. The patient is told to resist unnecessary movement but not to feel
    bound to one position. If necessary, the patient can readjust his or her
    position.
7. Finally, the therapist provides the patient with a rationale for relaxa-
    tion training. One could say that relaxation training will enable the
    patient to control various aspects of stress, such as muscle tension,
    visceral reactions, and negative thoughts. Those patients being pre-
    pared for chemotherapy can be informed that when in a relaxed state
    they will be able to control physiological reactions such as anticipatory
    nausea and vomiting in addition to emotional reactions such as anxi-
    ety. The patient can be told that relaxation produces a calming effect
    that helps to reduce the possibility of an upset stomach and, in addi-
    tion, helps distract one from the negative thoughts surrounding the
    process of chemotherapy. Cotanch (1983) and Carey & Burish (1988)
    have used similar explanations in their work treating patients with
    conditioned aversive reactions from chemotherapy.

A rating scale can be used to evaluate the patient's progress in learning
relaxation skills. The scale can range from 0 to 100 or 0 to 10 depending

on the patient's preference: 0 would signify no tension or anxiety, and 100 would signify the maximum. Patients can rate their anxiety and tension levels both before undergoing a relaxation exercise and as soon as it ends. The patient can employ the rating scale each time he or she engages in home practice, reporting the results to the therapist.

Further procedural points to remember include the following: Tell patients with contact lenses that they may wish to remove them so that they can keep their eyes closed without fear of irritation. Suggest to patients that they wear comfortable clothing for sessions during which relaxation training will take place. Have men either loosen or remove their neckties prior to commencement of the relaxation procedures.

Patients find it easier to learn relaxation when the therapist records the relaxation procedures on cassette tape for them to use at home. After the patient has practiced for several weeks, it is useful to tell him or her to start practicing without the tape every second or third home-practice session. This reinforces learning and gives patients confidence that they are capable of relaxing on their own. The importance of home practice is emphasized and reinforced. It is often helpful to devote several therapy sessions to relaxation training and practice.

Breathing Techniques. Diaphragmatic breathing is particularly effective as a relaxation technique in controlling visceral reactions, such as rapid heart rate, hyperventilation, excessive sweating, nausea, and vomiting. Relaxation can be produced by breathing slowly (approximately 8 seconds to complete a full breath, including both an inhalation and exhalation). During diaphragmatic breathing, the abdominal area rises during inhalation and flattens during exhalation.

A useful strategy in getting patients to understand what is meant by diaphragmatic breathing is to have them place one hand on their abdominal area and the other hand on their upper chest. If they are breathing correctly, only the abdominal area will rise. Another useful technique involves having the patient lie on a flat surface such as a couch and place a book or a box of tissues on his or her stomach. If the patient is breathing correctly, the book will rise during inhalation and descend during exhalation.

The therapist can help the patient learn to breathe more slowly by counting to four while the patient inhales and by using the same count to four as the patient exhales. If the patient cannot breathe that slowly, the therapist can modify the count to 6 or 7 seconds instead of 8. Prior to commencing breathing retraining, the therapist should assess the patient's breathing pattern. Is the patient already able to breathe diaphragmatically or is the patient a thoracic breather (i.e., uses the chest instead of the diaphragm)? How rapidly does the patient naturally breathe? Asking the patient to just breathe as he or she usually does, the therapist measures the breathing rate and uses it as a baseline. Using the concept of successive approximations (i.e., taking small steps in the right direction), the therapist systematically encourages the patient to breathe at gradually slower rates. For example, a patient who initially breathes at 14 breaths per minute may be encouraged to slow his or her breathing down to 12 breaths per minute. When successful, the goal could be set at ten and then eight breaths per minute.

Patients are also taught to breathe through their nose as opposed to engaging in mouth breathing. Breathing through one's mouth can lead to overbreathing, especially if one is anxious, which would then lead to hyperventilation and further anxiety.

Patients are encouraged to practice the breathing techniques twice a day for 2 minutes at a time. Most patients find it easier to initially practice breathing diaphragmatically when lying flat. Eventually most people can learn to breath diaphragmatically in sitting and standing positions as well.

Progressive Muscle Relaxation. Progressive muscle relaxation training as developed by Jacobson (1938) is a process by which the individual learns to relax by alternately tensing and relaxing the various muscles of the body. The reason why the patient is instructed to purposely tense a muscle and then to release the tension is to learn to discriminate between tension and relaxation. The patient will eventually learn to recognize feelings of tension and will then be able to relax by letting go of the tension. The patient is encouraged not to strain muscles while they are performing the tension phase. Only three-fourths tension is necessary. The patient is encouraged to practice the complete exercise twice a day for several weeks. When we first introduce progressive relaxation, we usually demonstrate the various steps of the procedure so that the patient knows exactly what to do. We find that doing the exercise with the patient helps him or her to feel more comfortable doing it in our presence. The following is a progressive-relaxation exercise based on Jacobson's (1938) technique, with some modifications by the present authors:

Make yourself comfortable. Your arms are at your sides, your fingers open, your eyes can be either open or closed during this first exercise, and your legs are not crossed. Once you feel comfortable with the exercise, you may want to close your eyes to obtain the maximum benefit of relaxation.

The exercise involves tightening your muscles, one group at a time. Then concentrating on the feeling of tension in a particular muscle group, then letting go and relaxing that muscle group. We will start with the feet and legs. Press your feet down flat as if you were pushing through the floor. Your toes are pressed together. This tightens your legs, your thighs, and your buttocks. Study the feeling of tension from tightening your muscles. Hold the tension, and now let go. Just relax. Feel that tension flow out. Concentrate on the muscles of your toes. Relax your toes. Relax the muscles of your legs. Feel the relaxation in your ankles, calves, and knees. Relax your thighs. Relax the muscles of your buttocks. Let the tension go. Feeling more relaxed.

Now the muscles of your abdomen. Tighten up your abdominal muscles. Study where you feel the tension. Hold it, and now relax. Feel the tension flow out, concentrate on the feeling, and relax the muscles of your abdomen. Just let go. Feeling more and more relaxed.

Now the muscles of your back. Arch your back and feel the tension. Feel the tension in the long muscles along the spine. Feel it, just hold it, and now let go. Let your back sink into the chair. Feel the relaxation spreading up and down your spine.

Now the muscles of your fingers and your arms and your shoulders. Make a tight fist with each hand. Make your arms stiff and straight, and raise them from the shoulder to about a 45-degree angle. Now feel the tension. You feel it in your fingers, your forearms, upper arms, and shoulders. Hold it, and now relax. Lower your arms and let them hang by your sides, fingers open. Feel the tension flow out. Concentrate on relaxing the muscles of your fingers. Just let them go. Relax your forearms. The muscles of your upper arms and shoulders, feeling more relaxed. No need to hold onto any tension.

Now the muscles between your shoulder blades and the muscles in your neck. Pull your shoulders back so your shoulder blades almost touch and at the same time arch your neck and point your chin to the ceiling. Feel the tension. Feel it in the back of the neck muscles. Tense, tense, and now let go. Feel that tension flow out. Relaxing the muscles between your shoulder blades. The muscles of your neck. No need to support your head, just allow the muscles to become loose and limp. Find a comfortable position for your head. Feeling so relaxed.

Now the muscles of the face. We will start with the muscles of your jaw and tongue. Clench your jaw. Keeping your jaw tight, push with your tongue against the back of your teeth. Tense, tense, and now relax. Just let the muscles go loose and limp. As you relax the muscles of your jaw, you may find that your lips and teeth part slightly. Tighten the upper parts of your face, close your eyes tight, feeling the tension around your eyes and at the bridge of your nose. Hold it, but do not strain it. Tense, tense, and now relax. Feel the tension flowing out. Relaxing the muscles around your eyes and the bridge of your nose. Feel the relaxation. Feeling more and more relaxed. Now tense your forehead by raising your eyebrows. Feel the tension in your forehead and scalp. Now let go and relax. Lower your eyebrows and feel your forehead becoming smooth, soft, and relaxed. Just let that happen as you feel more and more relaxed.

Now just allow yourself to breathe slowly and deeply and with each exhalation feel yourself becoming more and more relaxed. Just keep letting your body relax. Your whole body becoming calm and relaxed. With each exhalation, becoming more and more relaxed. With each exhalation, feeling the tension leaving and relaxation taking its place. Becoming more and more relaxed. Calm and relaxed.

"Letting Go" Relaxation. The next phase in learning muscle relaxation involves learning to let go of tension without first having to tense the muscles. As Goldfried and Davison (1976) point out, "letting go" relaxation is the next logical step in learning muscle relaxation. Having learned to let go after initially tensing, it is fairly easy and natural for the patient to simply let go of tension without tensing. After several weeks of practicing the Jacobson progressive-relaxation procedure, the patient will become more aware of tension and better able to eliminate it. A transcript of "letting go" relaxation based on the one developed by Goldfried and Davison (1976) follows:

Lie down, make yourself comfortable. Your arms are at your sides, your fingers open, your eyes are closed and your legs are not crossed.

You can begin by first focusing your attention on the muscles of your feet. Start letting go of any tension there. Relax your toes and feel the relaxation spreading throughout the muscles of your feet. Just relax. Now your legs. Let go of any tension in the muscles of your ankles, calves, knees, and thighs. Just allow the muscles to loosen up and relax. Each time you exhale see if you can let go further and further so that both of your legs are becoming loose and limp.

Now, let that feeling spread to the muscles of your stomach. Just let go of any tension in your stomach and allow your stomach to relax. Let the feeling spread into the muscles of your chest and as you allow the muscles of your stomach and chest to relax, you might find that your breathing becomes slower and deeper.

Now allow the feeling of relaxation to spread to your back muscles. Be aware of any tension there and let go of it. Let your back become loose and limp. Allow yourself to just sink back into the chair, feeling yourself becoming more and more relaxed.

Next, your arms. Notice any tension there and let go of it. Let both arms hang loose and limp, shoulders hanging comfortably, hands open, fingers apart, wrists limp. Feel the relaxation in your lower arms, upper arms, becoming more and more relaxed. All your limbs hanging loose and limp, just as if you were like a rag doll.

Let go of any tension in your neck. Find a comfortable position for your head so that you can relax your neck muscles. Now let your jaw hang slack in a relaxed position with your teeth slightly parted, lips slightly parted. If you allow your lips and teeth to part slightly, you may feel an immediate release of tension throughout the muscles of your face. Feel the relaxation in your cheeks, your forehead, the muscles around your eyes all becoming more and more relaxed. Just continue breathing slow and easy, allowing yourself to drift into deeper and deeper relaxation.

Mantra Meditation. A mantra is a pleasant sounding word such as "calm," "one," or "Om," which an individual repeats silently for the purpose of achieving a relaxed state. This technique can be used by itself or in combination with diaphragmatic breathing. The individual is instructed to spend anywhere from 2 to 20 minutes breathing slowly and diaphragmatically and with each exhalation repeating the mantra silently. The individual is advised not to be concerned if stray thoughts intrude and simply to let them pass and return to the mantra. In addition, the individual is told not to be concerned if he or she forgets to repeat the mantra. If this happens, the patient is instructed to just continue the process, coordinating the repeating of the mantra with each exhalation.

Relaxation Imagery. An important component of relaxation training is the use of imagery. Researchers have consistently found that imagery involving pleasant scenes enhances the effectiveness of other relaxation procedures in helping cancer patients cope with invasive medical procedures (Burish, Carey, Krozely, & Greco, 1987; Burish & Lyles, 1981; Carey & Burish, 1988; Cotanch & Strum, 1987).

The therapist and patient collaborate in developing an image. The patient can be asked to describe a specific place that he or she finds relaxing and enjoyable such as the beach. The patient is asked to describe the image using as many sense impressions as possible (visual, auditory, tactile-kinesthetic, olfactory, and gustatory). The therapist writes this information, which will be later used verbatim as part of a relaxation procedure.

Cognitive Restructuring

Cognitive restructuring procedures are used to help patients modify those attitudes, beliefs, and thoughts that cause excessive stress. We will now describe how the didactic method, the Socratic method, and the two-column method can be utilized for stress management.

The Didactic Method. As described in chapter 2, this method seeks through explanation to alter the patient's misconceptions and irrational beliefs. The didactic approach was taken with a patient who feared returning to work after being diagnosed as having cancer. Her fear was based on the belief that if she returned to work she would not be able to perform the duties of her position and would be a liability to the company. The therapist (W.D.G.) was didactic in that he directly clarified the patient's mistaken belief. The following dialogue took place between the patient and therapist:

Patient: I'm afraid to return to work because I'll fail.
Therapist: No. I don't believe you'll fail. You seem frightened of failure because you don't feel comfortable with your illness.
Patient: That's right. I won't be able to perform at the same level. Others will see me as incapable and I don't want to hurt the company.
Therapist: It's true, you may not be able to perform at the same level as

before, but your employer seems to want you to return. It seems that you are being harder on yourself and demanding more than others are demanding of you.

Patient: I should demand more. I don't want charity. Maybe it will be better if I just stay home and let the illness take its course.

Therapist: I know you're not incapable and you know that to be true. In addition, when was the last time you heard of your company giving charity? They obviously see you as capable or they wouldn't want you to return. Just don't expect yourself to be able to work as hard as you did before your cancer.

Patient: You're right. I know it's true. I'll go back to work and not expect as much of myself. I realize that what you're saying makes sense.

Therapist: Remember, you're not responsible for your disease. You can change the way you see yourself by taking the risk to see if my views about your company are correct. I think they are.

Patient: It's true, I was feeling responsible and I see now that I assume what others are feeling.

The intervention in this case involved getting the patient to see that it was not necessary for her to be as productive and demanding as she was in the past and that she would be happier and less stressed if she returned to work. She agreed to take the risk, and, indeed, she did experience a marked increase in happiness and her will to live as a result of resuming work.

The Socratic Method. As described in chapter 2, with the Socratic method, thought-provoking questions are asked by the therapist with the intent of getting the patient to reevaluate some of his or her self-defeating ideas and misperceptions. In contrast with the didactic method, where the therapist corrects the patient's faulty thinking, when using a Socratic approach the therapist helps the patient to arrive at the rational thought. If in the above example the therapist had taken a Socratic approach, the following dialogue could have taken place:

Patient: I'm afraid to return to work because I'll fail.

Therapist: What makes you say that?

Patient: Because I feel I'm unable to be as productive and people will be upset with my performance.

Therapist: Are you sure others will be unhappy with your performance or will you be unhappy with your performance?

Patient: That's true. I feel I should be like everyone else. I don't want charity.

Therapist: Do you think your boss expects you to be like everyone else?

Patient: Well, no.

Therapist: Do you believe he would ask you to return to work if he felt you were unable to perform your duties?

Patient: That's probably true. Knowing my boss I feel he would tell me to take the time to stay home if he felt I was incapable of working.

Therapist: So, is it true that you are being given charity or are you a valuable member of the company in which your services are needed?

Patient: I see what you're saying. I guess I'll go back. I'm sure I can do it.

As discussed in chapter 2, a therapist may combine or alternate between the Socratic and didactic methods of disputation. At the beginning of treatment, the therapist will usually have to be more didactic. However, once the patient learns the basics of cognitive therapy, the therapist can switch to a more Socratic style and place more responsibility on the patient. However, whenever a patient has difficulty in being more rational, despite the therapist's use of good reflective questions, the therapist should not delay in switching to a more didactic style.

The Two-column Method. This method is useful for helping patients to reevaluate self-defeating thoughts and can be used to construct coping self-statements. The coping statements can be used whenever the patient catches him or herself engaging in a self-defeating pattern of thinking. Coping self-statements can also be rehearsed during desensitization and stress-inoculation training (to be discussed later).

In presenting the two-column method, the therapist instructs the patient to divide a page into two columns and to write at the top of the page the stressful event being discussed. On the left side of the page the patient lists his or her irrational self-defeating thoughts. These self-defeating thoughts are identified through previous self-monitoring assignments or are uncovered during therapy sessions. In the other column, the patient lists a rational coping statement for each self-defeating thought. Most patients will need help in developing rational statements, although later in therapy they will be able to develop the statements on their own. They are encouraged to use the coping self-statements whenever they notice themselves reacting to anxiety-producing thoughts. At that point, they replace the negative self-defeating thoughts with the rational coping self-statements.

In Table 3.3 is an example of the two-column method using the dialogue from the patient above who was having difficulty getting back to work. Her coping self-statements were developed with the help of her therapist. First, the therapist would ask her if she could arrive at a rational statement. When she had difficulty in constructing rational statements the therapist offered more assistance by giving actual suggestions.

Table 3.3. Sample Two-Column Method
Situation: Patient Is Deciding About Returning To Work

Irrational Thoughts	Rational Statements
1. I'll fail if I go back to work.	1. I know my work. I'm still capable of performing my job.
2. I'll be a charity case.	2. My boss is not a person who would do that. He realizes that I'm capable.
3. I won't be able to work as hard as before and will be a liability to the company.	3. My boss knows I won't be able to work as hard, but it's okay. I'm capable and therefore the company won't lose anything.

IMAGERY REHEARSAL

Imagery is particularly useful because for most people vividly imagining a stressful event will evoke anxiety to almost the same degree as would occur from being in the real-life situation. Imagery provides the patient with an opportunity to practice coping with stressful events under supervised and safe conditions. Imagery is an important component in desensitization therapy and stress-inoculation training.

Desensitization

Systematic Desensitization, which was first developed by Wolpe (1958), was later refined by Goldfried who refers to his modification as coping desensitization (Goldfried, 1971; Goldfried & Davison, 1976). Meichenbaum (1977, 1985) has developed a similar approach which he calls stress-inoculation training.

Whereas Wolpe conceptualized desensitization in terms of counterconditioning, Goldfried and Meichenbaum have reconceptualized it as a method for teaching coping skills. In Goldfried and Meichenbaum's coping-skills approach, the patient is made aware of the external stressors in his or her life and the maladaptive self-defeating attitudes, beliefs, and thought patterns that produce and/or maintain feelings of anxiety. Stress-monitoring forms such as the one described earlier in the chapter can be used to identify these stressors and maladaptive thoughts. A list of the stressors (called a hierarchy) is developed. Each stress-inducing situation is identified and rank ordered from least to most anxiety producing. Each stressor can be rated by the patient on a Subjective Units of Discomfort Scale (SUDS) from 0 to 100, where 0 is no anxiety and 100 is the maximum amount possible.

Coping skills are then taught. Along with relaxation training, the patient is taught cognitive-restructuring techniques and is helped to develop a set of coping self-statements that can be used to replace the maladaptive self-defeating thoughts. The two-column method described earlier in the chapter is a simple procedure for producing coping self-statements.

After developing some proficiency with the coping skills, the patient is given preparation in coping with stressors. Prior to being asked to imagine any anxiety-producing situations, the patient is helped to achieve deep relaxation. While in the relaxed state, the patient is instructed to imagine each anxiety-producing situation. If the patient becomes anxious, he or she applies the various relaxation techniques and coping self-statements in reducing the anxiety. The items from the hierarchy are presented one at a time from least to most anxiety producing. During the imagery, the patient is presented with the least anxiety-producing item and, after experiencing success in reducing anxiety to that item, is then presented with the next. This process is continued until the patient successfully progresses through each item of the hierarchy. Finally, the patient is encouraged to apply these tools *in vivo* (i.e., real-life situations).

In Wolpe's (1958) original method of desensitization, patients were instructed to terminate imagining the scene as soon as they felt anxiety and to employ instead progressive relaxation in order to return to a more relaxed state. The current authors use the coping model developed by Goldfried (1971) in which the patient practices coping with the stressful situation. If a patient reports feeling anxious during the procedure, he or she is instructed to signal the therapist but to continue imagining the anxiety-producing scene while using the relaxation techniques and coping self-statements to reduce the anxiety. Several signaling procedures can be used. The patient may either raise his or her index finger to indicate the presence of anxiety or may use the SUDS scale and report the level of anxiety being experienced. We find it helpful to encourage the patient to strive for an acceptable SUDS level (such as 30) instead of expecting to achieve an unrealistic goal of 0 anxiety. If the patient is unable to reduce the anxiety to an acceptable level, then the patient is instructed to stop imagining the scene and to focus on reinducing relaxation. Once relaxation is reestablished, the item can once again be presented. The same procedure is followed with each hierarchy item.

If the therapist is careful in constructing a finely graded hierarchy, the desensitization will usually proceed smoothly. Desensitization is most effective when the therapist is careful not to proceed to a higher item on the hierarchy, like a 50 SUDS item, until a patient can deal with a 40 SUDS item. Care should be taken to proceed very slowly at the patient's pace, making sure that the patient feels in control and is not nauseous or anxious before proceeding to the next item.

A number of investigators have found relaxation and desensitization to be effective in controlling the adverse effects of chemotherapy (Burish et al., 1987; Burish & Lyles, 1981; Carey & Burish, 1987; Cotanch, 1983; Cotanch, Hockenberry, & Herman, 1985; Dahlquist et al., 1985; Hailey & White, 1983; Lyles, Burish, Krozely, & Oldham, 1982; Morrow, 1986; Morrow & Morrell, 1982; Redd, Andersen, & Minagawa, 1982; West & Piccionne, 1982; Zeltzer, Kellerman, Ellenberg, & Dash, 1983; and Zeltzer, LeBaron, & Zeltzer, 1984). Relaxation is effective when used with veteran chemotherapy patients, but will be more effective when introduced before chemotherapy has begun (Burish et al., 1987).

Helen, a patient who had a phobic reaction to chemotherapy, will be used as an example of desensitization. Helen's surgery was successful in removing a cancerous tumor and she was receiving chemotherapy as a precautionary measure. Midway through her chemotherapy program, she developed a conditioned aversive reaction. In addition to vomiting after receiving chemotherapy, she experienced anticipatory anxiety, nausea, and vomiting to many previously neutral stimuli. These stimuli were used to construct a hierarchy. Her hierarchy with SUDS ratings consisted of:

1. Walking into the admitting office — 20%
2. Sight of the nightgown used at the hospital — 30%
3. Suitcase used for hospital — 35%
4. Nurse calling to make appointment — 40%
5. The sight of the IV on the pole — 45%
6. Being in the hospital the night before receiving chemotherapy — 50%
7. The sight of the basin — 55%
8. Walking into the hospital room — 60%
9. Having to use the commode — 65%
10. The doctors bringing out the chemical vials — 70%
11. Waiting in the hospital room for the treatment to begin — 75%
12. Starting the IV — 80%
13. Anticipating getting symptoms from the chemotherapy — 82%
14. Vomiting after chemotherapy — 85%
15. Getting Parkinsonian symptoms from the chemotherapy — 90%
16. Recalling the second chemotherapy treatment which was the worst — 95%
17. Vomiting from the chemotherapy late at night — 98%
18. Shivering from the chemotherapy — 100%

In the above case, diaphragmatic breathing, "letting go" relaxation, relaxation imagery, and coping self-statements were used as part of desensitization. Helen's pleasant image was a beach in Hawaii. In addition to the diaphragmatic breathing, Helen found that recalling the smell of pineapple also reduced the nausea. Coping self-statements such as "You're going to be okay, this is helping you and giving you life" were used to control negative thoughts about the chemotherapy such as, "Oh my God, I will die, the drug is killing me." Desensitization was successful in completely eliminating the conditioned aversive reaction and helped to reduce the severity of Helen's side effects from the chemotherapy.

Desensitization is extremely flexible, and various modifications of this procedure are possible. This is illustrated by the following case. Carol was experiencing panic attacks during her radiation treatments. A careful assessment revealed that Carol had a long history of claustrophobia and was afraid of elevators, restaurants, buses, and trains. However, she experienced a higher level of anxiety during radiation treatments than in any of the other situations. Therefore, her desensitization hierarchy included items concerning elevators, restaurants, buses, and trains, which were presented first because they had lower anxiety ratings. Carol did not use coping self-statements because she preferred to use relaxation skills alone. Her desensitization was successful and enabled her to cope with the radiation therapy and to feel more comfortable in buses, trains, elevators, and restaurants. This case illustrates the importance of being flexible and doing a proper assessment.

Stress-Inoculation Training

There are situations where the use of a hierarchy is not needed or there is not enough time to develop one. Meichenbaum's (1977, 1985) modification of desensitization, stress-inoculation training, is particularly appropriate for such situations. In stress-inoculation training, the patient employs relaxation procedures and coping self-statements while mentally rehearsing how to cope with a specific stressful situation.

A stress-inoculation training procedure was employed in the case of a woman who underwent breast surgery. After surgery, she felt unattractive and embarrassed about sex, even though her husband was still interested in her sexually. The therapist and patient jointly developed several coping self-statements, such as "I am not ugly — I am still a pretty woman and my husband and I still can enjoy a satisfactory sex life. Even if we feel uncomfortable at first, we can work it out."

The patient already had been taught relaxation and was successful in using it for other stressful situations. She was therefore very receptive to applying it to her sexual anxiety. First, relaxation was induced using the "letting go" technique. Then the therapist instructed her to rehearse the coping self-statements while imagining herself talking to her husband about sex. After listening several times to a cassette tape of the procedure, she felt more relaxed and comfortable with approaching her husband.

SUMMARY

This chapter focused on stress-management principles, techniques, and applications for the treatment of anxiety and stress-related disorders. Stress-management techniques, such as relaxation training, cognitive restructuring, stress-inoculation training, and desensitization therapy were described, and their applications were illustrated through case examples. In the next chapter, we will discuss how stress management and other procedures can be used in the control of pain.

Chapter 4
Pain Control

Hypnosis and cognitive-behavior therapy can be used in the treatment of cancer patients with chronic pain, presurgical pain, and pain stemming from invasive medical procedures. There are several significant similarities between hypnosis and cognitive-behavior therapy. For example, relaxation and imagery are employed in both approaches. Because of their commonalities, hypnosis and cognitive-behavior therapy are very compatible and can be integrated for maximum effectiveness (Golden, 1983a; 1985; 1986; Golden, et al., 1987; Golden & Friedberg, 1986). There are also unique contributions from each approach. Cognitive-restructuring procedures are particularly effective in helping patients cope with pain. Hypnotic interventions, such as dissociation, hypnotic anesthesia, and hypnotic analgesia, are unique in their ability to eliminate pain for periods of time in moderately and highly hypnotizable patients.

Although the combination of hypnosis and cognitive-behavior therapy enhances the effectiveness of treatment for many cancer patients, there are some patients who are afraid of hypnosis (Hendler & Redd, 1986). Hypnosis is most effective when it is provided to individuals who have positive attitudes and expectations about it (Lazarus, 1973; Spanos & Barber, 1974, 1976). Typically, the patients who respond well to hypnosis are those who request it on their own or are enthusiastic after being informed that it is an available option.

TYPES OF CANCER PAIN

Cancer pain is a multidimensional phenomena and can involve physiological, perceptual, cognitive, emotional, behavioral, environmental, and interpersonal factors. It is therefore very important for assessment and treatment to also be multidimensional. Cancer pain can be subdivided on

46

the basis of whether it is chronic versus acute and disease-related versus treatment-related.

Acute Pain

Acute pain is characterized by a well-defined pattern of onset. It is time-limited, less than 6 months duration. Usually it is associated with both subjective and objective evidence of autonomic nervous system reactivity (Bonica, 1979; Foley, 1986). The patient will show signs of distress that can include increased heart rate, sweating, muscle tension, elevated blood pressure, and increased respiration (Jay, Elliott, & Varni, 1986; Sanders, 1979). Acute pain is most often exhibited in patients experiencing presurgical pain and treatment-related pain. Stress-management procedures and hypnosis are often effective with acute pain.

Chronic Pain

Pain is considered chronic when it persists for longer than 6 months. Patients with chronic pain are frequently depressed and often suffer from sleep disorders and loss of appetite. They are likely to be experiencing lifestyle changes where the pain affects work performance, recreation, and social activities. Chronic pain may be intermittent, intractable, or progressive.

Intermittent pain is similar to acute pain in that it is time-limited. However, intermittent pain is chronic in that it is recurring. Although varying in intensity, intractable pain is present most of the time. Often there is an adaptation of the autonomic nervous system so patients with intractable pain may exhibit less objective evidence of stress (Foley, 1986). However, depression may play a significant role and contribute to the patient's suffering.

Secondary gains may be operating in intermittent and intractable pain. The patient may be excused from responsibilities, may receive disability benefits, or receive increased attention from others. These secondary gains may reinforce dependency, helplessness, and even the intensity and frequency of the pain. In such cases, pain-reducing procedures alone are often not enough. Treatment needs to be multidimensional and address the various factors and issues involved.

Chronic progressive pain is often experienced by patients with metastatic cancer. Their pain becomes progressively more intense, frequent, and physically debilitating. Psychological factors, such as anxiety about dying and feelings of hopelessness, intensify the pain (Foley, 1986). Chronic progressive pain is so stressful that it becomes increasingly more difficult for a patient to keep up the effort required to apply pain-reducing techniques. However, secondary gains are rarely a factor when pain reaches this level. Patients are motivated to find relief and as long as they have the emotional and physical strength available they are usually cooperative. Treatment can then be focused mainly on pain relief by any and all employable measures. As anxiety is a prominent feature of this type of pain, stress-management procedures can provide some relief. Hypnotic interventions, such as dissociation, hypnotic anesthesia, and hypnotic analgesia, can be used to reduce some of the pain. But, because the pain is progressive and constant, it is not possible to totally eliminate it, regardless of the patient's motivation and hypnotic ability. At best, hypnosis and cognitive-behavior therapy are successful in reducing the intensity and duration of the pain. It is unrealistic to expect these techniques to replace medication. They are to be used in addition to whatever pain-reducing medications the patient requires.

Disease-related Versus Treatment-related Pain

Cancer pain may be further subdivided as being either disease-related or treatment-related (Bonica, 1980; Foley, 1979, 1986; Jay et al., 1986). Disease-related pain is the result of tumor involvement, either compression or infiltration of bone, nerve, or soft tissue. Treatment-related pain refers to the pain resulting from antitumor treatments, such as surgery, radiation therapy, and chemotherapy, as well as invasive diagnostic procedures, such as bone marrow aspirations and lumbar punctures.

Multidimensional Assessment of Cancer Pain

A number of factors are involved in the experience of pain. As pain is not just a physiological phenomena but can involve perceptual, cognitive, emotional, behavioral, interpersonal, and environmental factors, a multidimensional assessment is needed in order to determine which of these factors are operating in a given case. Then a comprehensive treatment plan can be developed which would include interventions for each relevant factor. A multidimensional treatment approach is particularly important in the treatment of chronic pain, which is more complex and difficult to treat than acute pain. The following classification will be useful as a guideline in conducting a multidimensional assessment.

Physiological Factors in Pain. According to the International Association for the Study of Pain (1979), pain involves unpleasant sensations "associated with actual or potential tissue damage." However, a purely physiological explanation of pain fails to account for phantom pain, where pain is felt in a missing limb, and fails to explain why people react differently to the same types of pain-inducing stimulation. It also fails to explain why hypnosis, acupuncture, and electrical stimulation reduce pain. According to the gate-control theory of pain (Melzack & Wall, 1965), neural mechanisms in the spinal cord act like a gate that can increase or decrease the flow of nerve impulses from the pain receptors. The gate-control mechanism can be influenced by the brain, which explains how the experience of pain can be modified by psychological factors.

Perceptual Factors in Pain. The perception of pain is greatly influenced by attention. Many patients with chronic pain become passive and focus on their pain. The more one focuses on pain, the more one is aware of it. Diverting one's attention away from the pain will lessen it and in some cases will result in a temporary absence of pain. A number of cognitive-behavioral and hypnotic interventions may block pain through distraction (McCaul & Malott, 1984; Redd, Jacobsen, Die-Trill, Dermatis, McEvoy, & Holland, 1987). Distraction from pain can be accomplished through externalization, which involves getting patients to focus their attention on external stimuli, such as listening to music, watching movies, playing with video games, or engaging in other tasks (Corah, Gale, & Illig, 1979; Farthing, Venturino, & Brown, 1984; Kolko & Rickard-Figueroa, 1985; Redd et al., 1987). Distraction can also occur through the use of imagery and other cognitive activities. Spanos and Barber (1974, 1976) have accumulated evidence supporting their view that hypnosis is effective to the degree to which the individual becomes absorbed in the imagery and suggestions that are part of the hypnotic procedure. Later in the chapter we will present a hypnotic-skills training program that enhances hypnotic responsiveness by teaching patients how to focus their attention and become absorbed in therapeutic imagery and suggestions.

Cognitive Factors in Pain. One of the best predictors of success in pain management is whether or not an individual catastrophizes about the pain (Turk, Meichenbaum, & Genest, 1983). Catastrophizers focus on and exaggerate their pain. The cognitive style of the catastrophizer interferes with his or her ability to use coping strategies for pain control (Spanos, Radtke-Bodorik, Ferguson, & Jones, 1979). Cognitive-restructuring procedures, which will be described later in the chapter, can be used to control catastrophic thinking (Ellis, 1962). The patient is taught to identify and alter the maladaptive thoughts that increase the patient's anxiety and pain. In addition, other cognitive coping techniques, such as distraction techniques and redefinitional strategies, which will be described later in the chapter, can be employed for pain relief.

Emotional Factors in Pain. As mentioned earlier, anxiety is often a component of the pain experience. A vicious circle can develop where pain causes anxiety and the anxiety intensifies the pain, which then leads to more anxiety. When stress-management procedures are effective in reducing pain, it is mainly because they interfere with this vicious circle.

Depression can result from the prolonged stress that is part of chronic pain. Patients with chronic pain often feel helpless and hopeless. The therapist should therefore evaluate the patient for the possibility of depression and, if needed, include interventions for depression when formulating a treatment plan.

Behavioral Factors in Pain. In general, with most types of pain, activity reduces pain; passivity intensifies it. There are several possible explanations as to why activity reduces pain. When patients are occupied, their attention is diverted away from their pain. Activity also reduces anxiety and depression, and may therefore break the vicious circles involving anxiety, depression, and pain. Physical activity may have the additional benefit of stimulating the production of beta endorphins, the body's natural pain reducers (Goldstein, 1973).

We have seen many instances where increasing the activity level of a cancer patient was particularly effective in reducing pain and depression. However, there are a number of cancer patients for whom physical activity is contraindicated. As pointed out by Cleeland and Tearnan (1986), some cancer patients experience pain only when they are active. Furthermore, physical activity may even be dangerous for patients with metastatic bone cancer. Physical activity could fracture their already compromised vertebrae. For these patients, more passive types of activity, such as reading, watching movies, and listening to music, can be considered instead.

Interpersonal and Environmental Factors in Pain. Interpersonal and environmental factors have been grouped together because they both have the potential for becoming reinforcers of pain, which are often referred to as "secondary gains." Although sympathy, attention, financial benefits, and being excused from responsibilities can reinforce pain, this is not always the case. Sympathy and attention from others may increase a patient's morale and motivate the patient to utilize pain-relief strategies. Some patients suffer in silence and need to be encouraged to talk about their pain. These patients often do not receive proper pain-control medication because they are afraid that they will inconvenience others or be perceived as "complainers." According to Marks and Sacher (1973), many cancer patients are undermedicated. With these patients, validation of their feelings is the proper therapeutic intervention. They need to be told it is appropriate for them to verbalize their feelings and ask for help, including asking for whatever medication they require.

Interpersonal and environmental factors should be suspected as sources of secondary gain when resistance to treatment is manifested by the patient. For example, the patient may fail to implement any of the pain-relief procedures, or may reject every technique claiming that they will not work. The therapist needs to address the resistance and assess whether or not secondary gains are the source. There may be other reasons why the patient resists or rejects help. Golden (1983b) has outlined the various types of resistances and other obstacles that may be encountered in cognitive-behavior therapy and has described various methods for overcoming them. For example, patients may give up prematurely or not try because they feel helpless and hopeless. In that case, the patient's depression also needs to be treated. Another obstacle to treatment could be that the patient catastrophizes and gives up too easily. In this case, cognitive-restructuring procedures, which will be described later in the chapter, could be utilized.

When secondary gains are involved, treatment will need to be directed toward modifying the contingencies that reinforce the pain. The therapist will probably need to involve family members and significant others who may be inadvertently reinforcing unhealthy behaviors. The therapist teaches them how unhealthy behaviors, such as helplessness, passivity, withdrawal, and catastrophizing, increase pain. They are also taught how to avoid reinforcing these behaviors and to reinforce instead healthy coping behaviors. For example, family members can be instructed to encourage the passive patient to be more active. Patients who catastrophize and complain excessively, to the point that it interferes with their ability to cope, can be advised to minimize discussing their pain with family members. The family members can be taught to praise the patient whenever he or she employs the various pain-reduction procedures. Family members will require support and reinforcement from the therapist in order for them to be able to make these changes. More will be said about family counseling in our chapter designated for that subject.

ASSESSMENT OF CANCER PAIN

Part of the assessment process involves evaluating the patient on the basis of the various factors described above. Not all, nor even most patients, will have all of the possible contributing factors. In addition to interviewing the patient, assessment can be made on the basis of input from physicians, nurses, family, behavioral observation, self-ratings, questionnaires and self-monitoring. Ideally what will emerge from the assessment process is a conceptualization of the patient's pain and the formulation of a treatment plan.

Questionnaires

One of the most widely used instruments for measuring pain is the Melzack-McGill Pain Questionnaire (Melzack, 1975). It measures pain intensity and also sensory, affective, and evaluative aspects of pain. Its main clinical purpose is to assess the amount of pain relief obtained from an intervention or set of interventions.

A short questionnaire developed specifically for cancer patients is the Wisconsin Brief Pain Inventory (BPI) (Daut, Cleeland, & Flannery, 1983). It takes only 10 minutes for a patient to complete the BPI. The BPI includes questions about pain intensity, antecedents that exacerbate the pain, and pain diminishers (i.e., strategies that the patient uses that are effective in reducing pain). Patients are asked how their pain affects their mood, work, sleep, activity, walking, pleasure, and social relations. The questionnaire also includes a shortened version of the Profile of Mood States (POMS) which is used for measuring mood disturbances. Daut et al. (1983) report that the BPI is both reliable and valid as a pretreatment and posttreatment measure.

Behavioral Observation

Behavioral observation provides the researcher or the clinician with an objective measure of pain and anxiety in children. The children are rated for how much distress they exhibit before and after receiving a pain-control intervention. The Observational Scale of Behavioral Distress (OSBD) (Jay & Elliot, 1984; Jay, Ozolins, Elliott, & Caldwell, 1983) and the Procedure Behavioral Rating Scale (PBRS) (Katz, Kellerman, & Siegel, 1980) were developed specifically for measuring distress in children with cancer who are undergoing invasive medical procedures. In these scales, the behaviors to be rated are operationally defined, so as to make it easy for independent observers to identify and score each sign of distress. The reader is referred to Katz et al. (1980) and Jay et al. (1983) for the complete scales and their scoring systems.

Katz et al. (1980) report that the PBRS can reliably differentiate between high- and low-anxious children. Jay et al. (1983) report that the OSBD is highly reliable and valid. One criticism of these scales is that they do not differentiate between pain and anxiety (Katz, Kellerman, & Siegel, 1981; Schacham & Daut, 1981). However, it is extremely difficult to distinguish between pain and anxiety when measuring acute pain through behavioral observation. Therefore, the term "behavioral distress" is appropriate as "a general term encompassing behaviors of negative affect, including anxiety, fear and pain" (Katz et al., 1981, p. 471).

For children, behavioral observation is more accurate as a measure of acute pain because it does not depend on introspection and verbal abilities that are required in self-ratings, questionnaires, and self-monitoring. Self-report measures are more appropriate for adults who do not exhibit the behavioral signs of distress that are observed in children.

Self-monitoring

In the previous chapter on stress management, self-monitoring was described in detail. Self-monitoring can aid the therapist in performing a functional analysis of a patient's pain. Antecedents such as events, actions, thoughts, and feelings that exacerbate or diminish pain can be identified. Self-monitoring also enables the therapist to measure pain in terms of its frequency, intensity, duration, and the amount of medication used, thus making it possible to monitor the patient's progress. For the majority of patients, pain-control procedures reduce rather than eliminate pain. Progress is usually gradual and may be very subtle, perhaps observable on only one measure, such as a reduction in the intensity or the duration of the pain. Many patients expect dramatic results from pain-reduction procedures. When their pain is not immediately and fully eliminated, they can become discouraged and give up. Self-monitoring provides the clinician with the data necessary to demonstrate to the patient that changes are occurring. A self-monitoring form such as the one in Table 4.1 can be given to patients. Depending on the patient and the situation, the form can be modified to include more or less details. Keep in mind that patients with advanced cancer are often too exhausted or too distracted to do much, if any, record keeping.

When monitoring the amount of medication used by a patient, the therapist should clarify that the goal is not to reduce the patient's medication. As pointed out by Cleeland and Tearnan (1986), the most significant difference between the treatment of pain in cancer patients and the treatment of non-life-threatening types of chronic pain is in terms of goals about medication. In treating other types of chronic pain, one goal is to have the patient eventually reduce or eliminate pain medication. However, the reduction of pain-reducing medication is not usually appropriate as a goal for patients with progressive malignant cancer. Cognitive-behavior therapy and hypnosis are to be viewed as adjunctive treatments and not as substitutes for pain-relieving medication. As the disease progresses, the patient will probably require more rather than less assistance in controlling pain. As mentioned earlier, patients often need to be taught to be more assertive in requesting effective dosages of medication because many cancer patients are undermedicated.

Table 4.1. Pain Log

Situation	Thoughts	Feelings	Actions	Pain Intensity (1–10)	Duration	Medication

COGNITIVE-BEHAVIORAL INTERVENTIONS

Relaxation Techniques

Relaxation techniques, as described in chapter 3, are effective in helping patients cope with pain. As discussed earlier in the chapter, anxiety is usually a component of acute pain and chronic progressive pain. People typically tense up and become anxious in response to pain, which then intensifies the pain. Relaxation procedures break this vicious circle.

Essentially, relaxation procedures are used for pain reduction in the same manner as they are used for reducing anxiety. The instructions and training procedures are the same as those described in detail in the chapter on stress management. The patient learns to use relaxation techniques as coping tools that can be applied whenever pain is experienced. Patients are advised to intervene as soon as they start to experience pain, so as to prevent the vicious circle that can develop if their anxiety is given a chance to spiral. They are advised that relaxation procedures do not usually totally eliminate pain. However, they can reduce at least some of the pain. Relaxation procedures can also be part of a larger treatment package for pain relief, such as the stress-inoculation program to be discussed later.

Distraction

Earlier in the chapter, perceptual factors as they influence pain were discussed. Patients can be given the following explanation:

"The more one focuses on pain, the more it becomes intensified. Therefore, you can reduce it by diverting your attention away from the pain."

Then, distraction techniques can be introduced. Distraction can be internal, for example, through daydreaming or the use of imagery, or be external, such as reading, listening to music, or watching movies. Some patients are more responsive to activities that get them to focus externally; whereas others are more responsive to imaginal distraction. Distraction is effective to the degree to which the patient is absorbed in the task. The degree of absorption will depend on the patient's level of interest in the task. Therefore, video games and stories involving superheroes will be effective with children. When music is used, it should be based on the patient's preferences. Classical music would probably not be effective with a rock-music fan and vice versa. In using imagery for the purpose of distraction, the images may involve pleasant relaxing scenes but, as research shows, they could be neutral or even involve anger (McCaul & Malott, 1984). Patients are helped to construct detailed images that they will find interesting and absorbing.

During therapy sessions, patients who are experiencing pain practice applying various distraction techniques to discover which ones are most effective. They can report on the effectiveness of each technique in reducing pain by rating their pain before and after implementing each technique. Patients preparing for painful invasive medical procedures can be taught a package of techniques to be tried when they are needed.

Reviews of the research literature conclude that distraction is somewhat effective in reducing mild to moderate pain (McCaul & Malott, 1984; Tan, 1982) but is more effective when used as part of a treatment package such as stress-inoculation training (Turk et al., 1983).

Redefinitional Strategies

Cognitive relabeling, or reframing as it is often called, and objectification are redefinitional strategies. With each of these techniques, the patient's interpretation of the pain is the focus of change. In sharp contrast with distraction, the patient using objectification focuses on the specific sensations of the pain, analyzing and describing them in objective terms. The patient describes the size and location and rates the intensity of the pain. With cognitive relabeling, the meaning of the pain is transformed. For example, cognitive relabeling was employed with a patient who interpreted his postsurgical pain as "a sign of impending death." His anxiety and some of his pain were reduced when, following the advice of his therapist, he relabeled the pain as "part of the recovery process from surgery."

In a review of the literature comparing distraction and redefinitional strategies, McCaul and Malott (1984) report that distraction is more effective with milder pain, whereas redefinition is effective with intense and prolonged pain. Patients can be advised to combine strategies, using distraction and relaxation when their pain is mild and switching to redefinitional strategies if the pain intensifies or is prolonged.

Individual differences are additional factors to be considered. Distraction is more effective with "repressors" than it is with "sensitizers" (McCaul & Malott, 1984). Repressors can be defined as individuals who tend to cope with stress by avoiding it. Sensitizers are receptive to learning about the stressors they will encounter. One way of differentiating repressors from sensitizers is to ask patients whether they prefer to know or not know as much as possible about a medical procedure before undergoing it. The repressors would rather not know.

Cognitive Restructuring

As mentioned earlier in the chapter, maladaptive thoughts can interfere with an individual's ability to cope with pain. Instead of employing coping strategies, patients who catastrophize dwell on their pain and magnify it. Catastrophic thoughts, such as "I can't stand this pain," "It will never go away," and "It's just going to get worse and worse until it kills me," will elevate the patient's anxiety and intensify the pain. Patients who catastrophize are often unable to benefit from hypnosis and cognitive-behavior therapy unless some type of cognitive restructuring is employed. Other self-defeating patterns of thought that interfere with an individual's ability to utilize pain-control interventions include helplessness and hopelessness ("I can't do it, it's hopeless") and self-deprecation ("I'm too weak, I'm such a coward").

The first step in cognitive restructuring is to educate the patient about how one's thoughts affect the experience of pain. The next step is to identify the patient's specific self-defeating thoughts. Frequently, these thoughts are verbalized by the patient in the form of complaints, such as "It's too terrible, I can't stand it." The therapist is sympathetic but explains how focusing on the "awfulness" of the pain makes it worse and then explains how coping self-statements can be employed. The self-monitoring form (see Figure 4.1) can also be used to pinpoint the thoughts, feelings, and actions that intensify the pain. During the week, the patient uses the self-monitoring form in between therapy sessions to record this information, which is reviewed at the beginning of each therapy session. Then the patient and therapist work together to construct coping self-statements as alternatives to the maladaptive thoughts.

Another method for identifying catastrophic thoughts involves the experiential method, which is used during therapy sessions. Whenever a patient is having trouble employing a pain-control procedure, the therapist can ask the patient what he or she was thinking at the time that the pain-control technique was being implemented. Often, the difficulty is that the patient is unable to focus on the intervention because he or she is dwelling on the pain and catastrophizing about it. Rather than abandon that particular pain-control technique, the therapist can help the patient identify the catastrophic thoughts and then proceed with cognitive restructuring. The patient may then be able to employ the pain-control intervention.

The Two-column Method. The two-column method described in chapters 2 and 3 is a cognitive-restructuring procedure that can be used to modify maladaptive thoughts. The patient's maladaptive thoughts are written in the left-hand column and coping self-statements are written in the right-hand column. The patient and therapist collaborate to construct the coping self-statements. Table 4.2 provides an example of the two-column method with Martin, who suffered chronic pain as a result of metastatic bone cancer. At first, relaxation and hypnosis were impossible to implement because Martin repeatedly opened his eyes, was restless, and grimaced throughout the procedures. Attempts to employ various distraction and redefinitional strategies also failed. The therapist (W.L.G.) helped Martin to realize that he focused on the pain and catastrophized instead of concentrating on the therapist's instructions. Several maladaptive thought patterns were identified: "Nothing is going to work. Why bother?" "The pain is too intense," "If medication didn't help, this psycho-shit certainly won't," "I'm such a coward. I should be able to stand this pain," "But it's unbearable."

The therapist took special care to be empathic and nonconfrontational so Martin would not think he was being criticized. After the therapist helped Martin to identify his self-defeating thoughts, the following dialogue took place:

Therapist: You're experiencing a great deal of pain and you're being too hard on yourself. Most people would have trouble coping with this type of pain. It's no wonder that you're having trouble keeping your mind focused on therapy. But maybe we can do something about it. We might not be able to eliminate the pain but maybe you can get at least some relief.

Patient: How? It seems so hopeless.

Table 4.2. Sample Two-column Method for Pain Control

Negative Thoughts	Coping Self-statements
1. Nothing is going to work. Why bother?	1. Keep trying.
2. The pain is too intense.	2. Just reduce it to a manageable level. Use brief relaxation such as slow deep breathing and think "calm" or use some pleasant imagery.
3. If medication didn't help this "psycho-shit" certainly won't.	3. This can work. Let's see what works.
4. I'm such a coward. I should be able to stand this pain.	4. I'm not a coward. This type of pain is difficult to cope with.
5. It's unbearable.	5. It's intense but I can be strong. I've survived. I can cope with it.

Therapist: I understand why you feel that way. We've tried a lot of different techniques and so far none have helped. But it seems to me that the main problem is that the pain keeps distracting you.

Patient: Right.

Therapist: Sometimes what helps when the pain is that bad is to use what we call coping self-statements. They don't necessarily reduce the pain but they can make it easier to handle. Would you like me to show you what I mean?

Patient: Yeah, I guess I have nothing to lose.

The therapist wrote Martin's self-defeating thoughts in the left-hand column of a page folded in half (Table 4.2). The therapist then proceeded to enlist Martin's aid in constructing the coping self-statements.

Therapist: Thoughts such as "Nothing is going to work, why bother" are what we call self-fulfilling prophecies. I know it feels like it's true. That's understandable. You've tried a lot and so far nothing has helped. But, let's see if we can come up with a more constructive way of looking at the situation. Can you think of a different way of looking at it or would you like me to make a suggestion?

Patient: What about "Keep trying?"

Therapist: That sounds fine. The important thing is to counteract the negative thought with a more constructive one. Let's try another one. The next one on your list is "The pain is too intense." I have a few suggestions for this one. We find that with intense pain the more you focus on how intense it is, the more intense it becomes. The best strategy is to focus on something else other than the pain. But don't expect to eliminate it. That might be unrealistic. A more realistic goal is to reduce it to a more manageable level.

Patient: Sometimes those distraction methods you taught me did reduce the pain a little, but I thought it should have been more.

Therapist: Maybe a combination of techniques will work better. How about reminding yourself to just reduce it to a manageable level and use some slow deep breathing and distraction, like thinking about something else other than the pain?

Patient: Yeah, I have nothing to lose.

Therapist: The idea is, whenever you catch yourself thinking a negative thought, replace the negative thought with a coping thought. Then use the other techniques such as the deep breathing and distraction. And keep in mind they may not reduce the pain each and every time. Use them to reduce the pain as much as possible, and even when they don't reduce pain you can still use them to cope with it better.

Martin and his therapist proceeded with the cognitive restructuring until a full set of coping self-statements was developed. Martin combined the coping self-statements with some brief relaxation (deep breathing along with the word "calm" and various pleasant and distracting images). Martin did experience some pain relief despite progression of his illness. According to Martin, what was most helpful was learning to not focus and dwell on how bad the pain felt.

Stress-Inoculation Training

Stress-inoculation training (Meichenbaum, 1977, 1985) was described in the previous chapter for stress management. It has also been used for pain management (Turk et al., 1983). Stress-inoculation training has been found to be effective for adults in treating several clinical pain syndromes (see Turner & Chapman, 1982) as well as with children undergoing painful medical treatments for burn injuries (Elliott & Olson, 1983). Several studies have demonstrated that a multicomponent program, based on stress-inoculation training, is effective in reducing distress in children with cancer undergoing painful medical procedures, such as bone marrow aspirations (BMAs) (Jay, Elliott, Katz, & Siegel, 1987; Jay, Elliott, Ozolins, Olson, & Pruitt, 1985).

As applied to the treatment of pain in adults, stress-inoculation training consists of several stages. First, the patient is educated about pain. The Melzack and Wall (1965) gate-control theory, described at the beginning of the chapter, is typically used as the explanation. In our work with cancer patients, we emphasize that perceptual, cognitive, emotional, behavioral, and interpersonal factors affect physical pain. Patients are then taught coping skills such as relaxation procedures, distraction, redefinitional strategies, and the use of coping self-statements for pain management. All of these techniques are taught; however, each patient decides which coping techniques he or she will employ. Experimentation is encouraged. Patients try various strategies and determine for themselves which ones are effective.

Patients with chronic pain can apply the various coping techniques during therapy sessions. The therapist teaches a technique, guides the patient in its application and helps the patient to evaluate its effectiveness. The patient develops a set of coping techniques that he or she then applies whenever they are needed.

Several modifications are possible in preparing patients for painful medical procedures such as surgery, BMAs, lumbar punctures, and other invasive diagnostic and treatment procedures. Adult patients can practice the various coping techniques while imagining themselves experiencing the various steps involved in the painful medical procedure. Behavior rehearsal has been used to prepare pediatric cancer patients for BMAs and lumbar punctures (Jay et al., 1985, 1987). First, the child plays doctor and gives a doll the BMA or lumbar puncture using real medical equipment. The doll is "coached" by the child to use the relaxation breathing techniques. Then the therapist role plays being the patient and models the breathing exercises and various other coping techniques such as coping self-statements and emotive imagery, which is imagery involving the child's favorite superhero (to be discussed in the next chapter). Emotive imagery (Lazarus & Abramovitz, 1962) is more appropriate than relaxation imagery for reducing distress in children. Children relate more to fantasies about their favorite television and cartoon characters. These stories absorb their attention more than would descriptions of peaceful serene scenes.

Another modification of stress-inoculation training by Jay et al. (1985, 1987) is the use of modeling films for teaching coping skills to children. A 12-minute film entitled "Joy Gets a Bone Marrow and Spinal Tap" depicts a 6-year-old leukemic patient modeling various coping techniques. The film also provides information about the specific steps of each procedure. The film is based on Meichenbaum's (1971) finding that "coping" models who initially manifest anxiety before successfully coping are more effective than "mastery" models who show no fear. The child in the film first describes her fearful thoughts and distress, then receives cognitive-behavioral treatment from a psychologist and finally successfully copes with the BMA and spinal-tap procedures. The Jay et al. (1985, 1987) program also utilizes small trophies as rewards for lying still and using the breathing exercises during the procedures. A different method of positive reinforcement is used in stress-inoculation programs for adults. Adults are encouraged to use self-reinforcement (i.e., praising themselves for having successfully coped).

Operant Methods

Fordyce (1976) has developed operant conditioning programs for treating chronic pain. Operant programs are based on the assumption that "pain behavior" is learned and can be extinguished and replaced with "healthy behavior." The patient's family and health-care workers are instructed to ignore pain behaviors such as excessive crying, complaining, grimacing, and helplessness and to reward, praise, and encourage healthy behaviors. A wide variety of chronic pain syndromes have been treated in structured inpatient operant programs. However, operant conditioning has rarely been applied in a systematic manner to the treatment of cancer patients with chronic pain.

A case reported by Redd (1982) provides an illustration of operant conditioning as applied to a hospitalized cancer patient. The presenting problems of the patient, a 64-year-old male in the final stages of cancer, were his crying, moaning, and yelling. He was already receiving high dosages of morphine for his pain. Nevertheless, he spent 60% of his awake time crying, moaning, and yelling. The intervention involved time-out, where attention was withdrawn when the patient engaged in the "pain behaviors" and social reinforcement when he did not. This intervention was selected based on the observation that the patient exhibited greater distress when others were present. After 10 days of the operant program, the patient's crying and other signs of distress ceased.

We would recommend trying alternative treatments before considering operant conditioning techniques such as the time-out procedure described above. As pointed out by Turner and Chapman (1982), the limitations of the operant approach are that cognitive processes associated with chronic pain are ignored. The goal of operant programs is to modify pain behaviors and the experiential aspects of pain are largely ignored. As described earlier, family counseling is an alternative way of modifying reinforcement contingencies that may be providing the patient with secondary gains. Furthermore, the focus in cognitive-behavior therapy is on a collaborative relationship with the patient, where the emphasis is on teaching the patient self-control procedures. Operant conditioning can be considered if a collaborative approach and/or family therapy is impossible or fails. Redd reports that, in the case described above, other medical methods had failed and other psychological interventions, such as relaxation and hypnosis, were considered but were rejected because of the patient's extreme agitated state.

HYPNOSIS

There are a number of therapists who have reported success in employing hypnosis for relieving cancer pain (Ament, 1982; Araoz, 1983; Barber, 1978; Barber & Gitelson, 1980; DeBetz & Sunnen, 1985; Erickson, 1959, 1966, 1983; Gardner & Olness, 1981; Hilgard & Hilgard, 1975; Hockenberry & Bologna-Vaughn, 1985; LaBaw, Holton, Tewell, & Eccles, 1975;

Margolis, 1983, 1986; Olness, 1981; Sacerdote, 1962, 1970; Shapiro, 1983; Zeltzer, 1980). In several clinical studies, hypnosis was found to be effective in reducing cancer pain (Butler, 1954; Cangello, 1961; Lea, Ware, & Monroe, 1960; Speigel, 1985; Speigel & Bloom, 1983) and was effective in helping children and adolescents cope with painful medical procedures (Hilgard & LeBaron, 1982, 1984; Kellerman, Zeltzer, Ellenberg, & Dash, 1983; Zelter, Kellerman, Ellenberg, Barbour, Dash, & Rigler, 1980; Zeltzer & LeBaron, 1982).

Stages of Hypnotherapy

Hypnotherapy consists of several stages:

1. Preparation of the patient for treatment
2. Hypnotic induction
3. Deepening of the hypnosis
4. Utilization of hypnosis for therapeutic purposes
5. Termination of hypnosis.

Preparation includes an assessment of the patient's problem, educating the patient about hypnosis, and the establishment of rapport. Many hypnotherapists also test the patient's hypnotic susceptibility. In the cognitive-behavioral approach, hypnotic susceptibility is usually not tested. Instead, a skills-oriented approach is taken whereby the patient is taught how to be responsive to hypnotic suggestion (Golden et al., 1987; Golden & Friedberg, 1986). But before initiating hypnotic-skills training, the patient's misconceptions are clarified.

Many patients come to therapy with misconceptions about hypnosis. Many expect to be passive and for the therapist to control them and remove their symptoms through direct suggestion. As a result of the way that hypnosis is depicted in the media, many patients expect to be asleep or unconscious. Common fears are that the hypnotized individual might not awaken from the trance, that hypnosis may weaken the mind, or that the hypnotized individual will be out of control. Another set of common misconceptions revolve around the belief that in order to be hypnotized, one has to be gullible, unintelligent, weak minded, or mentally disturbed. The therapist explains that hypnosis is safe and that researchers have failed to find any negative trait associated with hypnotic ability. The therapist can clarify other misconceptions with the following explanation of hypnosis:

"Hypnosis requires a collaborative effort between the therapist and patient. In order for hypnotherapy to be effective, you have to cooperate. Hypnosis is not sleep. You will not be unconscious. You will be in a pleasant, relaxed state and you will be fully in control."

Hypnotic-skills Training

We have found that by using hypnotic-skills training, almost all of our patients have been able to learn to use hypnosis, at least to some degree. The following is a transcript of hypnotic skills training adapted from Golden et al. (1987):

> *In order for you to learn to respond to suggestions for pain control, it is important that you first learn to respond to simple suggestions. Therefore, we are going to go through a series of exercises that are designed to help you learn how to respond to simple hypnotic suggestions. Hypnosis is not magical, nor is it something that happens to you. It requires your cooperation and participation. Hypnosis is a skill. Therefore, everyone can learn to respond and with practice you can get better at it. The skill is in being able to think and imagine along with suggestion. Hypnosis involves concentrating on thoughts and images that are consistent with the goals of a suggestion. For example, if your goal is relaxation, imagining a pleasant fantasy such as a country, mountain, or beach scene would help you to become relaxed. Likewise, you can also create relaxation with your thoughts or what can be called self-suggestions. In the case of relaxation, you could give yourself suggestions such as "My whole body is beginning to relax. My arms and legs are relaxing . . . beginning to relax more and more. The relaxation is spreading." Using pain control as another example, if you wanted to create anesthesia you would use thoughts and fantasies that would produce numbness. You could imagine that you were receiving an injection of Novocain and suggest to yourself, "My hand is becoming numb, I'm feeling less and less sensation. I'm starting to feel a rubbery feeling." You would continue the imaging and repeat these suggestions until you got the desired effect. Not only is it important to concentrate on the thoughts and fantasies that will produce the desired result, but it is also important to block out negative thoughts and fantasies that might interfere with your ability to respond to suggestion. If a person who is attempting to create a feeling of numbness focuses on thoughts that are incompatible with anesthesia (such as concentrating on the pain or thinking, "This will never work; I really didn't receive an injection of Novocain"), he or she will not obtain the desired results. There are several techniques you can use to block out these negative thoughts.*

Focusing

Simply focusing your attention and concentration on thoughts and fantasies that are consistent with your goals will usually be sufficient to obtain a successful response to suggestion. This method allows you to distract your attention from negative thoughts that would otherwise interfere with your concentration.

Thought Stopping

There are several thought-stopping techniques. First, think to yourself the word "Stop" whenever negative thoughts intrude into your consciousness. Second, after thinking "Stop," focus again on the thoughts and fantasies that are related to your goal. Each time a negative thought pops into your mind repeat the procedure. Some people find thought stoppage to be most effective when they imagine a traffic stop sign while thinking the word "Stop."

Letting Go of Negative Thoughts and Fantasies

Some people are able to "let go" of negative thoughts and do not need to use thought stoppage. Letting go refers to letting a thought pass through your mind instead of holding onto it and dwelling upon it. Occasionally, we all have negative and bizarre thoughts. If we are not alarmed by the presence of these thoughts and fantasies, and hence do not focus on them, our stream of consciousness will eventually flow to other thoughts. So if negative thoughts intrude, just let them pass and return to the thoughts and fantasies that will produce the desired results.

Now you are ready to apply these strategies to several exercises, so that you can discover which techniques work for you. You do not have to respond to all of the suggestions in these exercises in order to be a good hypnotic subject. As long as you are able to respond in some way to some suggestions, you will be capable of experiencing hypnosis.

Exercise #1 — Hand Heaviness

The goal of the hand-heaviness exercise is to create a feeling of heaviness in your arm. Before you begin, think of something that would be so heavy that you would eventually be forced to put it down. Make use of relevant experiences from your life. Some images that others have found helpful include: holding a shopping bag full of heavy books or groceries, lifting a barbell weight, trying to lift a piece of furniture, holding a bowling ball, and holding a huge book — like a dictionary — in the palm of your hand. You want to imagine holding something heavy which, if real, would make your arm tired and cause you to lower it.

Once you have selected your fantasy for producing hand heaviness, sit back in your chair and close your eyes. Most people can image better with their eyes closed. Hold both arms out in front of you, palms up. Keep your arms straight and parallel to one another. Imagine that you are supporting something very heavy with your dominant hand and arm.

Whatever you choose as your fantasy for heaviness, use as many of your senses as possible to imagine it. See it, its shape, its color, its size. Feel it. Recall the feeling of heaviness you experienced when you actually held or lifted the object.

In addition to using imagery, give yourself suggestions, such as, "My arm is feeling heavy, the muscles are getting tired, fatigued. I feel the strain in the muscles. My arm is feeling so heavy that I can't keep it up. I feel the weight pulling my arm down, down." Use your own words to suggest heaviness and lowering of the arm. It is important that you work with the suggestion by imagining an appropriate fantasy and thinking the appropriate thoughts. Block out any thoughts that are incompatible with the suggestions. Use focusing, thought stoppage, or the letting-go technique on any negative, competing thoughts. Imagine your arm getting so tired that it begins to drop lower and lower, until you can no longer keep the arm up, and you let it drop.

Exercise #2 — Hand Levitation

Think of something that would be consistent with developing a feeling of lightness in one hand. Some common images are of a large helium balloon under the palm of your hand; several helium balloons tied around your wrist; your hand is a balloon being pumped up with helium; your hand is a piece of metal being drawn upward by the magnetic force of your head, which is a huge electromagnet; and your arm is being lifted by a series of ropes and pulleys that are being manipulated by you or someone else. Feel free to use your imagination in creating your own fantasies and suggestions. As the goal is hand levitation, use strategies that will result in such strong feelings of lightness that your hand and arm lift up.

When you are ready to begin, close your eyes and extend your arms straight out in front of you. Use as many senses as possible to imagine your fantasy. If you are using a balloon image, picture its shape, size, and color. Feel its texture and buoyancy. Recall how balloons have felt to you in the past.

In order to make one of your hands feel lighter than the other, give yourself suggestions of lightness, such as, "I feel the lightness in the palm of my hand and throughout my arm. That arm is feeling lighter than the other. I feel slight movement in my fingers. I feel my hand lifting. The arm is lifting higher and higher, lifting up. . . . " Create your own suggestions in your own words. Imagine the balloon lifting up, rising into the air, and finally moving upward toward your face. Repeat the suggestions as many times as needed in order to create feelings of lightness and hand levitation. Give yourself time to respond. Remember to block out any intrusive thoughts that would interfere with the goals of the exercise.

Exercise #3 — Arm Catalepsy

The arm catalepsy exercise provides you with another opportunity to practice self-hypnotic skills. The goal of this exercise is to temporarily make your arm stiff and rigid. Think of something that would be consistent with your arm becoming rigid and immobile. Some people imagine their arm in a cast or a splint. Others imagine that their arms are bars of steel or are made of wood. Use your imagination and feel free to create your own fantasy.

First, make a tight fist and hold your arm out straight, stiff and rigid. Close your eyes and imagine your fantasy. Block out any interfering thoughts. While continuing to fantasize that your arm is immobile and telling yourself that it is immobile and cannot be bent, try to bend it. As long as you are absorbed in fantasies and thoughts *consistent with arm rigidity, you will have difficulty bending your arm. Once you stop imagining your arm as rigid, and you tell yourself you can bend it, you will in fact be able to move your arm easily.*

Hypnotic Induction

Two hypnotic-induction procedures, the relaxation method and hand levitation, will be described. The relaxation method is very similar to the "letting go" relaxation procedure described in the previous chapter on stress management. Most patients respond very well to it and therapists find it to be the easiest induction to implement. However, patients who responded well to the hand levitation exercise during the hypnotic-skills training are good candidates for the hand-levitation procedure. As in the case of stress-management procedures, cassette tapes of the hypnotic procedures can be recorded for home use. Readers interested in employing other hypnotic-induction procedures may consult Golden et al. (1987).

Hypnotic Relaxation. Various relaxation techniques such as slow deep breathing, pleasant imagery, and suggestions of relaxation can be employed for inducing hypnosis. As described in the previous chapter on stress management, we have our patients construct images that they find relaxing rather than using standardized images. The following procedure (from Golden et al., 1987) can be modified to be consistent with the personal preferences of the patient:

> *You can close your eyes and find a comfortable relaxed position. Let your body go limp and let yourself sink into the chair.*
>
> *Let your breathing start to slow down so that you are breathing slowly and deeply, a comfortable relaxed breathing pattern, where you are breathing in slowly and breathing out slowly . . . a comfortable rhythmic breathing pattern. . . .*
>
> *And as you continue to breathe slowly and deeply, your whole body will become relaxed . . . starting with your arms and legs. Feel your arms and legs starting to relax. Arms and legs hanging loose and limp, just as if you were a rag doll. Hands open, fingers apart, wrists loose and limp. Feel the relaxation spreading up and down your arms, all the way up to your shoulders. Just let your shoulders hang comfortably. Feel the relaxation spreading.*
>
> *And your legs, hanging loose and limp. Feel the relaxation spreading all the way down to your toes. Feel your toes and feet relax as you let your toes spread apart. Feel the relaxation in your ankles, calves, knees, and thighs. Both legs becoming more and more relaxed.*
>
> *Notice that with each exhalation you can feel yourself becoming more relaxed. Feel the relaxation spread with each exhalation. Breathing slow and deep. And with each exhalation feel yourself sinking into the chair more and more, into a deep relaxation.*

Feel the relaxation spreading to your back and neck. Just let your back go loose and limp. Feel yourself sinking into the chair even more, so that you are not holding yourself together. You're letting the chair support your body. Letting your neck be supported by the chair. Feeling the relaxation spreading, spreading to your stomach muscles, spreading throughout your body. Let your jaw hang slack, teeth slightly parted, and feel the relaxation spreading to your facial muscles, permeating your body. Feeling more and more relaxed. Continuing to breathe slowly and deeply and feeling more and more relaxed.

And to deepen your relaxation, you can imagine your peaceful relaxing scene, the one we discussed before. Imagine it as clearly and as vividly as you can, what it looks like . . . what you would see if you were there now looking out and enjoying the scenery . . . what you would hear . . . what you would feel . . . what you would smell . . . or taste . . . just keep on imagining that peaceful scene . . . just keep on imagining that peaceful scene, continuing to breathe slowly and deeply and feeling yourself becoming even more relaxed. Arms and legs, more relaxed. Shoulders hanging comfortably. Back and neck loose and limp. Jaw hanging slack. Facial muscles, smooth and relaxed. Stomach muscles, relaxed. All the muscles of your body, relaxed and your mind feeling calm and peaceful. As you continue to imagine that peaceful, serene scene and continue to breathe slowly and deeply, you become more and more relaxed.

Hand Levitation. As mentioned earlier, the hand-levitation exercise from the skills-training program is also useful as a hypnotic induction. The therapist utilizes the same image that was effective in producing lightness during the training. The patient is instructed to close his or her eyes and the therapist describes the image (such as the helium balloons tied to the wrist):

When you are ready to begin, close your eyes and let each hand rest gently on your legs. Use the same image that worked for you before when we did the hand-levitation exercise. (Therapist describes image.) Focus on one of your hands and be aware of whatever sensations develop in your hand . . . . Notice the difference between your hands . . . . Notice how one hand is starting to feel lighter than the other . . . . Feel the lightness spreading . . . spreading throughout your hand . . . spreading to your wrist . . . and your arm . . . . Your hand is getting lighter . . . and lighter . . . . Your arm is getting lighter . . . getting lighter . . . so much lighter than your other arm . . . . Soon it will feel so light that your arm will start to lift . . . . Feeling so light that it feels like lifting, like floating, light and buoyant. (The therapist repeats suggestions of lightness until some movement is detected and then proceeds.)

Your hand is so light that it begins to move . . . starts to lift . . . lifting . . . rising . . . feeling so light and buoyant . . . lifting higher . . . and higher . . . rising . . . lifting up . . . rising up . . . higher and higher.

Suggestions of movement are repeated until the upward movement of the arm stops. Then the therapist may shift to suggestions for deepening hypnosis or suggestions for producing hypnotic anesthesia or analgesia (to be described in the next sections).

Deepening Techniques

Several methods can be used to deepen hypnosis. Pleasant imagery and suggestions of relaxation, warmth, and heaviness can be used to deepen hypnosis. Other methods, such as the stairway image and the counting technique, can also be employed for deepening. The reader may refer to Golden et al. (1987) for additional deepening techniques.

The Stairway Image. The therapist asks the patient to imagine him or herself walking down a stairway and suggests that with each step, the patient is entering a deeper state of hypnosis. Some patients prefer elevators or escalators instead of the stairway. Some patients prefer going up instead of going down. Some patients like to control the depth of the hypnosis, increasing it or decreasing it by pushing the buttons of the elevator or going down the stairway only as far as they wish. The therapist should honor these preferences and involve the patient in the choice and design of the deepening technique. The following is offered as a guideline to be altered in accordance with each patient's preferences:

> *And to enter a deeper state of hypnosis, imagine walking down a stairway . . . a very pleasant stairway. . . . Imagine walking down at a very relaxed, comfortable pace. . . . Each step you take helps you to enter a deeper state of hypnosis, and you can go as deep as you want by going down as many steps as you want. . . . Imagine each step you take . . . taking you deeper . . . every step helps you to feel more relaxed . . . calmer . . . more deeply relaxed . . . deeper . . . each step . . . taking you deeper. . . . You're walking down at a very relaxed pace . . . feeling more comfortable, more relaxed with each step . . . down . . . deeper and deeper.*

Counting Technique. The therapist counts upward from 1 to 10 or downward from 10 to 1 and suggests that with each count the patient will enter a deeper state of hypnosis:

> *And now to enter a deeper state of hypnosis, I will count from 1 to 10. And with each count you will become more relaxed, entering a deeper state of hypnosis with each count. . . . 1 — With each count, becoming more relaxed . . .2 — Each count helps you to go deeper . . . 3 — Letting yourself go as deep as you want . . . 4 — Continuing to breathe slowly and deeply, and becoming more relaxed with each exhalation . . . with each count . . . 5 — Becoming more relaxed . . . 6 — Feel yourself becoming more calm . . . more relaxed . . . breathing slowly and deeply . . . 7 — More and more relaxed . . . 8 — Deeper and deeper . . . 9 — Feeling yourself going even deeper . . . 10 — In a deep, relaxed hypnotic state, feeling so relaxed.*

Utilization of Hypnosis

Hypnotic relaxation can produce some pain relief. However, as Hilgard and Hilgard (1975) point out, additional benefits can be obtained through hypnotic methods which produce analgesic and anesthetic effects. Several of the techniques will now be described. The reader interested in learning about other hypnotic techniques for pain relief can consult Crasilneck and Hall (1975), Erickson (1966, 1983), Golden et al. (1987), Hilgard and Hilgard (1975), Hilgard and LeBaron (1984) and Sacerdote (1970).

Hypnotic Analgesia and Anesthesia. In using hypnotic anesthesia, care should be taken not to mask pain that requires medical attention. This is usually not a problem because hypnotic anesthesia typically wears off after a period of time and only provides temporary relief. Nevertheless, we recommend that hypnosis should be used for pain relief only after a proper medical diagnosis has been made. We ask our patients to obtain permission from their physicians before we treat them with hypnosis. In addition, we remain in contact with their physicians.

In hypnotic anesthesia, the individual experiences an absence of sensation in a designated part of the body. In hypnotic analgesia, the effect is less dramatic and there is only a dulling of sensation. Essentially the same hypnotic procedure is used to produce anesthesia and analgesia. The patients who are most responsive to hypnosis will be capable of experiencing anesthesia in response to suggestions of numbness. Most individuals are only able to experience analgesia.

There are patients who are capable of experiencing anesthesia and analgesia through suggestion alone. However, most patients expect a hypnotic-induction procedure to precede the hypnotic suggestions. Therefore, we typically first employ one of the various hypnotic-induction procedures and use one or several deepening techniques before giving suggestions for pain relief.

Suggestion and imagery can be used to produce anesthesia and analgesia. Patients can be asked to recall the feeling of Novocain or imagine an anesthetic lotion applied to the painful area. Usually the words "pain" and "painful" are avoided as they may cause the patient to focus on the pain rather than sensations of numbness.

A method we have found effective in facilitating hypnotic anesthesia and analgesia is to divide the procedure into a series of steps. The therapist can proceed at the patient's pace, allowing enough time for each step to be experienced. As mentioned earlier, a hypnotic induction and one or more deepening techniques are usually employed prior to giving the following suggestions for anesthesia/analgesia. The wording can be modified to be consistent with the personal preferences of the patient:

In this hypnotic state your mind is receptive to therapeutic suggestions that will help you to feel better.

The first step is to imagine that your fingers are becoming numb. You can imagine that you have just used a pleasant anesthetic cream on the fingers of one of your hands and it is producing pleasant sensations. . . . Notice whatever sensations are produced. . . . You might be aware of a feeling of numbness in your fingertips . . . or a tingling sensation. . . . Just note whatever change in sensation you experience . . . and let me know when you experience the change by gently nodding your head. There's no need to speak, just nod your head and then I'll know to proceed . . .(patient nods).

And now the sensations of numbness will spread to the rest of your hand. Your fingers are becoming more numb and the numbness spreads to your hand . . . and when you feel your hand starting to become numb, let me know by nodding your head . . . (patient nods).

And now your hand will become more numb. Feeling less and less. . . . Becoming more and more numb. . . . And now you can transfer the numbness to your (designated area). You can now gently stroke your (designated area) and start to feel the numbness spreading from your fingertips to your (designated area). Gently stroking and feeling soothing sensations spreading from your fingertips to your (designated area). . . . And as soon as you experience the sensations spreading, let me know by nodding your head . . . (patient nods).

Feeling the numbness spreading and creating a very soothing, pleasant feeling. And whenever you wish to recreate this pleasant soothing numbness, you will be able to experience it by listening to the tape recording, or by using self-hypnosis, going through the same steps . . . imagining the anesthetic cream . . . the feeling of numbness in your fingertips and then your hand becoming numb. . . . And then transferring the numbness.

Dissociative Techniques. Dissociation occurs when certain aspects of one's experience are separated or "split off" from the rest of one's consciousness (Hilgard, 1979). This occurs in everyday life when an individual becomes so absorbed in reading a novel or watching a movie that he or she becomes less aware of other events in the environment. In terms of pain control, dissociation is the mechanism operating when a soldier is unaware of his wound until after the battle is over. Dissociation is also exhibited in athletes who are so absorbed in their sport that they are temporarily oblivious to any injuries they sustain during an event.

Hypnotic anesthesia and analgesia entail a dissociation from painful sensations (Hilgard, 1979). Dissociation can also be produced through other hypnotic interventions, some of which can be very dramatic. One technique consists of suggestions that the patient imagine his or her mind leaving the body. Usually only very good subjects can experience what feels like an out-of-body experience. However, most patients are capable of experiencing dissociation to some degree. After first inducing hypnosis and using several deepening techniques, the therapist can use the following suggestions to produce dissociation:

And in this deep state of hypnosis you can feel yourself drifting off, drifting off, and feeling detached, as if your mind were leaving your body.

Imagine yourself leaving your body and floating . . . floating. Looking down from above. Observing your body with a sense of curiosity. Feeling detached, as if you were watching someone else. You know it's you, but you feel detached . . . and more calm . . . feeling in control.

Often it helps to combine dissociation with imagery. The therapist can have the patient imagine leaving his or her body and going on a mental trip or back in time to a pleasant memory. Imagery can also be used to produce dissociation. Most patients experience at least some pain relief from imagery either as a result of dissociation or distraction.

When using imagery for dissociation, first the therapist and patient construct an image. It could be a relaxation scene or an image of some absorbing activity, such as the patient imagining him or herself skiing, swimming or horseback riding. After hypnosis is induced and the image is described, the following can be suggested:

As you continue to imagine (therapist mentions image), you can allow yourself to drift off . . . drifting off into a deep, deep, hypnotic state and feeling as if you were there now. Imagine being there now. (Therapist describes image again.) Becoming less aware of your surroundings, less aware of yourself.

Suggestions for Modifying Sensations. After hypnosis is induced, direct suggestions can be given that create soothing sensations to compete with pain. In addition to numbness, suggestions of warmth, coolness, or tingling can be given, depending on the preferences of the patient. Some patients associate coolness with pain relief; others prefer warmth. If a patient experiences the pain as a "burning" sensation, then suggestions of coolness would compete with, and reduce, the pain.

Sensory suggestions are usually most effective when combined with imagery. So, if a patient prefers warmth, then using a beach scene with "the warmth of the sun" will be more effective than merely suggesting that the patient will experience warmth. The imagery can involve color changes. The patient can be asked, "If your pain had a color, what color would it be?" One patient described his burning sensation as "red hot." The imagery incorporated the "burning red pain" as the starting point. Then it was suggested, while the patient was in a relaxed hypnotic state, that he imagine the color changing and the pain cooling off with each exhalation, turning orange, then yellow, and finally a cool white. The patient, who failed to respond to other hypnotic interventions such as dissociation and anesthesia, was able to successfully reduce his pain with the "color cooling" technique.

Termination of Hypnosis

There are several methods for terminating hypnosis. One is the counting method, where the therapist simply counts to a specified number, giving the patient suggestions such as the following:

Now you can start to return to the alert state. I'm going to count from 1 to 5, and at the count of 5 you will be wide awake, alert, and refreshed. 1 . . . I'm counting slowly so you can experience a comfortable transition from the hypnotic state to the wide awake, alert state. 2 . . . slowly starting to return to the wide awake state. 3 . . . 4 . . . starting to move a little. 5 . . . starting to open your eyes . . . relaxed, refreshed and wide awake.

Another method is to allow the patient to proceed at his or her own pace by suggesting the following:

Now you can start to return to the wide-awake state. Take your time, and proceed at a pace that's comfortable for you. Allow a comfortable transition, so that you proceed slowly. . . . And when you're ready, you can open your eyes, relaxed, refreshed, and wide awake.

Self-hypnosis

Patients can use tape recordings of the hypnotic procedures at home and also during invasive medical procedures. However, there are certain medical facilities where patients cannot bring their tape players. In these situations, self-hypnosis can be employed as a coping tool.

There are several methods of teaching patients self-hypnosis. Cassette tapes provide patients with the opportunity to have enough exposure to the hypnotic procedures so that eventually they are able to repeat them on their own without the tapes. Patients can also be given self-hypnosis scripts to memorize. The reader can consult Golden et al. (1987) for a set of self-hypnosis scripts and additional instructional material on self-hypnosis.

A posthypnotic cue provides another alternative method for teaching self-hypnosis. The patient is given a posthypnotic suggestion that enables him or her to enter self-hypnosis upon a given signal. The therapist arranges in advance with the patient what will be the signal. Any thought, image, or action can serve as a posthypnotic cue. We often use a method based on a technique described by Salter (1941). The following suggestion is given while the patient is in a relaxed hypnotic state:

Whenever you wish to enter hypnosis you will be able to do so by taking five, long, slow, deep breaths. With each exhalation, you will become more and more relaxed, so that by the fifth exhalation, you will be in a very pleasant, relaxed hypnotic state, similar to what you are experiencing right now. You will then be able to deepen the hypnosis by continuing to breathe slowly and deeply. You can also use your pleasant image to deepen the relaxation. And while in this relaxed hypnotic state you will be able to give yourself therapeutic suggestions, which will help you feel better and more in control. And when you wish to return to the fully alert, wide-awake state, all you have to do is count to 5 and suggest that by the time you reach the count of 5, you will be wide awake. Then you can open your eyes, feeling relaxed, refreshed, and wide awake.

CASE EXAMPLE

Tom's case will now be presented as an example of the use of hypnosis and cognitive-behavior therapy in the treatment of chronic pain. Tom's oncologist informed the therapist (W.L.G.) that Tom had an advanced case of cancer and predicted that he would probably only have 3 to 6 months to live. Nevertheless, the oncologist recommended that Tom return to work and exercise if he felt up to it. The oncologist gave the same information to the family, but they encouraged Tom to remain in bed. Tom sought psychological help for controlling his abdominal pain, insomnia, and lack of appetite. He wanted to be able to lead a more active life and return to work. He was receiving pain-relief medication but wanted to try additional methods of pain reduction.

Tom reported that when he was more active he experienced less pain and felt less depressed. Tom's wife expressed her fear that Tom's condition would deteriorate if he did not remain in bed. The therapist and the oncologist reassured her that activity was not harmful to Tom. The therapist also explained that when cancer patients are active, they enjoy a better quality of life and seem to live longer.

Tom was taught various cognitive-behavioral and hypnotic procedures for the treatment of pain, anxiety, and depression. He was responsive to all of the relaxation techniques described in the previous chapter on stress management. The quality of his sleep improved as a result of his practicing relaxation at bedtime. The time-projection technique described in the chapter on depression was used to help elevate his mood. Using the time-projection technique, he would imagine himself in the future, feeling better, scuba diving, working, traveling, and playing tennis. Activities such as mild exercise, swimming, doing chores, and visiting friends were encouraged. These activities significantly reduced Tom's depression and some of his pain.

Tom was enthusiastic about hypnosis, but hypnotic anesthesia and analgesia were not attempted because Tom thought they were "unrealistic." However, he was receptive to other dissociative techniques. He was able to identify several events in his life where he experienced some form of dissociation naturally and spontaneously. For example, when driving his car, he often found, as many people do, that he could become so absorbed in daydreaming that he felt as though the car was driving itself on "automatic pilot." Tom's previous experiences with dissociation helped him to experience it through hypnosis. While in a relaxed hypnotic state, he would imagine his favorite images: a beach scene, where he would "drift off listening to the sound of the surf," and a scuba-diving scene where he would become absorbed in the "beautiful iridescent colors" and movement of tropical fish. Dissociation was effective in helping Tom to get through moments when the pain was intense. For example, he used hypnotic relaxation and dissociation to go back to sleep when he awakened in pain. Hypnosis was also effective in helping Tom regain his appetite. While in a relaxed hypnotic state, images of his favorite foods were described along with suggestions that he would enjoy their taste and be able to eat more.

Cognitive restructuring was also employed. Through self-monitoring, Tom was able to identify several automatic thoughts that accompanied his pain, such as, "Something is very wrong, the end is here." He found that he catastrophized whenever he experienced an intensification of his pain. He would then become very anxious. Tom, with the help of the therapist, developed several coping self-statements, such as, "I've been through this before, it's nothing new, it will pass." These coping self-statements were effective in reducing his anxiety enough to enable him to employ the other techniques for pain reduction.

Tom continued to feel some pain. However, he could reduce its intensity to the point where he was able to enjoy life. He eventually returned to work and received a promotion before his death, which occurred 2½ years after his diagnosis of terminal cancer.

Chapter 5
Working With Children

Children have traditionally been referred to mental health practitioners because of some impending problem, behavioral disorder, family problem, school problem, or something which is disturbing the child to the point that normal day-to-day functioning is impaired. More recently, children are also being referred to mental health practitioners to learn to cope with chronic illnesses such as cancer or leukemia. Fortunately, cancer in children is rare and the prognosis has improved remarkably since 1962 with approximately 60% of children diagnosed with cancer expected to reach long-term remission now (Morris-Jones, 1987).

With specific types of cancer, survival rates tabulated in 1989 by St. Jude Children's Research Hospital in Memphis revealed that the survival rate of acute lymphocytic leukemia is up from 0% to 60%, Ewing's sarcoma up from 5% to 60%, Hodgkin's disease from 50% to 90%, retinoblastoma from 75% to 90%, and osteosarcoma is up from 20% to 60% (Bombeck, 1989).

Even though cancer remains the most common cause of death in children between 1 and 14 years old (Lansdown & Goldman, 1988), we have seen that progress in the field of pediatric oncology has dramatically raised the survival rate of childhood malignancy (Hammond, 1982). Because of the increasing survival rate of children with cancer, there is a greater need for services for these children. In many instances, the children do not understand what is happening to their bodies. They become angry at having to have chemotherapy or radiation therapy. They become angry at having their typical daily routine altered for constant hospital visits. They become embarrassed by the side effects of both chemotherapy and radiation treatment. Often they have difficulty coping with the world around them. It is the role of the mental health practitioner to help these children develop effective coping strategies for dealing with their illness.

PREPARING THE CHILD FOR THERAPY

It is important for the therapist to be properly organized and ready for the child to begin therapy. It is advisable for the therapist to spend a session (or two if necessary) with the parents before the child is seen in order to obtain background information.

Initial Consultation With Parents

The therapist meets with the parents of the child to obtain background information and also to provide support and any other psychological assistance that may be required. Maguire, Comaroff, Ramsell, and Morris-Jones (1979) point out that psychological support is often needed by the family members of the child with cancer. As will be explained in further detail in chapter 6, the family members experience intense emotional changes and need a means for coping with these feelings in a more rational manner. Family therapy is an important part of the child's treatment plan, as it continually offers the parents various tools and techniques for coping with many different situations that can arise during the child's treatment.

The initial consultation enables the therapist to obtain information about the child and the family as well as about the child's typical behavioral patterns and development. In some cases, the parents even spend two or three sessions with the therapist before the therapist sees the child. These sessions enable the therapist to do a complete assessment of the child and to develop a good working relationship with the parents. During these sessions, the therapist explains the need and importance of therapy for children with cancer. Spinetta and Maloney (1975) found that children with cancer experience progressively more anxiety as the disease progresses and that their anxiety also increases with each chemotherapy treatment. This increase in anxiety makes these children increasingly more prone to psychological problems as time goes on (Morrisey, 1963). In addition, children undergoing medical treatments for cancer must spend certain amounts of time away from their parents, which produces additional anxiety. Lansky and Gendel (1978) observed extreme separation anxiety coupled with regressive behavior in children with malignancies. Most parents realize the importance of psychological treatment and are cooperative.

One of the most common questions that parents ask the therapist is, "How do I explain you to my child?" One way to prepare a child is to advise the parents to say the therapist is a "talking doctor" who helps people with their feelings. It is important for the therapist to present him or herself differently than regular medical doctors, because children associate pain, hurt, crying, and discomfort with medical treatment. Some of the major complications of medical cancer treatment are physical discomfort, pain, weakness, and illness (Levine & Hersh, 1982). When told that they are going to see another doctor, children usually resist and sometimes become emotionally upset. The therapist presents him or herself as a nonpainful person.

Important Considerations Prior to Initial Session With the Child

Usually most children are somewhat tentative at their first session. The therapy situation is frightening to them and beyond their comprehension when they first begin treatment. The younger children (ages 4–7) usually want to have their mother or father come into the therapy room for security. Allowing either a parent, or even both parents, to come in with the child usually helps reduce the child's anxiety. Younger children often take a while before they feel comfortable with the therapist. Sometimes, special efforts on the part of the therapist are required. For example, one of the authors (D.M.R.) treated a 4 ½-year-old girl with a brain tumor who refused to come into the therapy room alone, so her mother came in with her. However, once inside with her mother, the child refused to talk with the therapist. The session was spent with the mother answering all of the questions. At the end of the session, the mother mentioned that the child loved stuffed animals. At the next session, the therapist was well-prepared with a dozen stuffed animals. Again the child refused to come in alone, so her mother accompanied her inside the therapy room. However, once inside the room, this time the child brightened up when she saw all of the stuffed animals. The therapist held a stuffed animal and made believe the stuffed animal was talking. The child responded to any questions asked of her by the stuffed animal, and gradually became comfortable enough to allow her mother to leave the room. After the session, she did in fact begin to talk with the therapist alone.

In many cases, the child has already begun chemotherapy or radiation therapy treatments prior to seeing the therapist. Children undergoing cancer treatment experience a number of bodily changes, such as hair loss, a change in complexion which sometimes results in their skin appearing chalky, weight loss, or sometimes even weight gain, as a result of the treatment (Van Dongen-Melman & Sanders-Woudstra, 1986). One of the major side effects of both chemotherapy and radiation therapy is the feeling of nausea. This feeling often stops the child from eating and this results in weight loss. Once chemotherapy and radiation therapy end, the nauseous feelings seem to disappear and children tend to regain weight

back to their normal weight level. We have also noticed that both chemotherapy and radiation therapy tend to make the child's complexion appear
to have a chalky tone. It should not come as any surprise if the child enters
the office wearing a hat or some head covering. Underneath the hat, the
child has probably begun to lose hair or may even be bald.

Care is to be taken to avoid letting the child's sickly appearance cause
any change in the therapist's greeting. Children are very sensitive to the
way other people look at them. They become very self-conscious and tend
to pick up cues very quickly from other people. The therapist should
present him or herself as a very friendly, warm, caring person as quickly
as possible. Children will respond in a most positive manner to this type
of greeting. Children feel most comfortable in a warm environment. They
begin to relax and quickly develop trust in the therapist. Usually, if a child
is comfortable enough to come into the therapy room without a parent,
this is a good indicator that the therapist has made a positive initial impres-
sion on the child.

The Initial Session

Initial sessions are quite important as they can set the stage for what will
happen later on in therapy sessions. The initial session is primarily used
as an information-gathering, get-acquainted session. Rapport can be established fairly quickly with a child in the first session if the session is kept
very light and filled with things that are humorous. Children respond very
positively to humor and fun. If the therapy room is filled with play toys,
funny posters, and cheery pictures it can have a most positive effect. It is
essential that the therapist address the child in a very warm, comfortable,
open manner while asking essential questions and assessing the child's
ability and level of communication. Typical questions involve age, family,
school, siblings, and friends. The following is a sample of what happened
during an initial session with a 6-year-old diagnosed as having cancer of
the eye orbit. He had already begun chemotherapy treatments.

Therapist: Hi, you're Barry, aren't you?
Patient: (Smiling) Yes.
Therapist: I'm Dave. Let me guess how old you are.
Patient: Okay.
Therapist: I'll bet that you are 16.
Patient: No (laughing), guess again.
Therapist: 12 years old.
Patient: No. (more laughing)
Therapist: How about 9 years old?
Patient: Nope!
Therapist: Well, then how old are you?

Patient: 6 years old.

Therapist: Wow! I would have never guessed your age, are you sure you are only 6?

Patient: Yes, I am.

Therapist: You sure are a big boy. How would you like to come into my office and talk to me a little? I have some great things to play with inside.

Patient: Sure.

The session continued very successfully. Barry was eager to see the office and play with some of the toys. He responded to all of the questions without any problems. He even asked a few questions of his own.

EVOCATIVE TECHNIQUES

Evocative techniques help children to express their perceptions, thoughts, and feelings. They can be used by the therapist for assessment and can also be employed for producing therapeutic change. After evoking the child's thoughts and feelings, the therapist can intervene and teach the child to cope more effectively. The different techniques described in this section are the ones we have found most easily adaptable and useful for working with children.

Play Therapy

A number of various play-therapy techniques can be used to elicit and assess a child's feelings about his or her illness. Children are most familiar with play. It is something that they have been doing ever since they can remember in their short lives. Play is usually associated with fun and happiness and can usually be done anywhere. We have found that play therapy does more than occupy children. It reduces uncertainty by providing play that is familiar, a welcome relief after all the strange sights, sounds, and bodily discomforts that children with cancer experience.

Lansdown and Goldman (1988) found that play therapy can also help prepare children for procedures and events like hair loss. Children have the opportunity during play therapy to express their feelings while playing and making believe they are at the hospital or receiving their medical treatments. The therapist can use stuffed animals, dolls, or even stick figures to represent someone who is sick as well as someone treating the sick person. During games such as these, children often express their own thoughts and feelings concerning treatment and side effects. Within the context of play therapy, they can talk about their feelings in a nonthreatening, supportive environment. The therapist can have a supply of stuffed animals, dolls, paper, pencils, and crayons, as well as toy figures of doctors, nurses, parents, and children for play therapy.

Picture Drawing

Children respond very positively to drawing. It is usually a skill they have previously utilized. In fact, there is really no incorrect way to draw. We have found that children respond quickly to a stack of plain paper and colored pencils. They seem to be very eager to draw something on the paper. The initial drawing is usually a self-portrait. Children love to draw themselves doing any number of different things, such as playing with a pet, playing with a friend, being with their family, or just by themselves. This self-portrait enables the therapist to understand how the child sees him or herself with respect to the illness. The therapist can then ask questions about the self-portrait and learn more information about the child. Other suggested drawings include the family, the chemotherapy or radiation room at the hospital, the hospital itself, the doctor's office, or even their classroom at school.

The drawings are an excellent way for the therapist to learn about the child's thoughts and feelings concerning the illness. Meichenbaum (1977) has described how Thematic Apperception Test (TAT)-like pictures can be employed to tap internal dialogues of children. Children are asked to tell what other children in the pictures are thinking and feeling and what the child in the picture can do to handle a given situation.

We have extended Meichenbaum's technique to children's drawings and have also used them to prepare children for future treatments or special situations that they may encounter. For example, an 8-year-old with a malignant tumor was about to begin radiation therapy. His parents mentioned that he was very anxious about the radiation treatment. The therapist (D.M.R.) began by having him draw pictures of the hospital and then pictures of the radiation treatment room with all of the equipment. He drew the doctors, the nurses, and finally he drew himself in the room. While the drawing continued, the therapist talked to him about his thoughts and feelings concerning the treatment. He revealed that all the equipment and machinery frightened him. The therapist explained why the equipment was there, what its purpose was and why it looked so scary. In addition, they talked about the radiation therapy and how it would help him get better. The child was then able to draw himself receiving the radiation therapy and not being scared of it. His final drawing was of himself leaving the hospital feeling well with a smile on his face.

The Use of Toy Blocks

Children love to create things with Lego-type blocks. Initially they are encouraged to play without a purpose. The therapist gives a great deal of praise for anything that is created. The therapist can use the blocks later to help the child confront situations and feelings that the child is avoiding. For example, hospitalizations usually elicit a high degree of distress and anxiety in children (Bozeman, Orbach, & Sutherland, 1955; Hoffman & Futterman, 1971; Natterson & Knudson, 1960). Nevertheless, children are often reluctant to talk about the hospital experience. The blocks can make it easier for a child to talk about his or her experiences, thoughts, and feelings. The blocks can be used to build a hospital. The Lego people can be used as doctors, nurses, and other children, as well as support staff. The therapist can orchestrate the scenario to assess the child's thoughts and feelings about the hospital experience. Both therapist and child work on building the hospital and placing the Lego people in the situation. During this play time, the therapist can ask questions of the child about his or her thoughts, feelings, and experiences. For example, Steven, a 7-year-old boy with leukemia, was very receptive to using the building blocks. He and the therapist worked on building the hospital. Steven created a Lego bus filled with children on their way to the hospital for medicine. Steven told the therapist that one of the children had diarrhea on the bus because he was nervous about going to the hospital. He also said that some of the other children were nervous as well. When asked about himself, Steven replied that he also got nervous and sometimes his stomach hurt from the treatment that he got at the hospital. By using the blocks, the therapist was able to elicit Steven's thoughts and feelings about the hospital and was then able to provide a way of teaching Steven to cope with them.

COGNITIVE-BEHAVIORAL INTERVENTIONS

As has been mentioned in earlier chapters, cognitive-behavior therapy techniques and procedures help adult patients to develop more rational thoughts and effective behaviors for coping with difficult situations. Cognitive restructuring, behavioral rehearsal, imagery, and relaxation procedures are all techniques that have been used effectively with adult patients to produce both cognitive and behavioral changes. These techniques can be modified for use with children. This section will describe some of the ways these techniques can be applied to children to help them cope more effectively with their illness and medical treatments.

Behavior Rehearsal

Throughout the history of cognitive-behavior therapy, therapists have relied on the use of behavior rehearsal (i.e., role playing) to help patients learn new patterns of responding to familiar situations. Through the use of role playing, patients may be presented with real-life situations in the safety of the therapy room. Both patient and therapist can work on the specific issues concerning a situation and help get the patient prepared to cope with a given situation in a more rational manner. Goldfried and Davison (1976) outline four general steps of behavior rehearsal. Step 1 involves the preparation of the patient in terms of having the patient recognize the need for learning a new behavior pattern. Step 2 involves the selection of the patient's problem situations. Step 3 is the actual role-playing phase. And step 4 is the carrying out of new role behaviors in real-life situations. We have adapted the use of role playing to our work with children.

It has been our experience that children with cancer face many new situations because of their illness and medical treatments. Role playing is an excellent way for the therapist to assess a child's thoughts and feelings about situations such as the child's medical treatment or school. The therapy room can be used to recreate situations such as doctor's visits, hospital visits, or people's reactions to the child whose appearance has changed. After evoking a child's thoughts and feelings through role playing, the therapist can then construct an appropriate treatment plan in order to help the child cope with the situation.

Stephanie, a 13-year-old with a malignant tumor, had to see several different specialists for her medical treatment. She revealed that she felt increasingly anxious with each new doctor. She had to tell each doctor about her particular case over and over again. She felt upset because she did not like discussing her medical history. She also did not like doctors because they usually made her feel some type of pain. Both Stephanie and her therapist worked on role playing in the therapy room. On some occasions, Stephanie was the doctor and asked the questions. The therapist was the patient and responded like a patient. On other occasions, Stephanie was somebody else with a different type of illness, and the therapist was the doctor. Through this process, she learned the importance of asking questions from the doctor's position and she also learned to respond in a calmer, more relaxed manner to the doctor's questions.

Cognitive Restructuring

Several different methods of cognitive restructuring were previously described: the didactic method, the Socratic method, self-statement modification, and the two-column method. Our experience has been that the most practical cognitive restructuring technique for children is the use of coping self-statements. A didactic approach can be taken with children in order to teach them how to develop and utilize coping self-statements. The idea is to keep it short and simple when working with children.

Coping Self-statements. The following example illustrates how coping self-statements may be introduced to children. During one of his therapy sessions, Jimmy, an 8-year-old with a malignant tumor, wanted to go outside for a walk. Jimmy was in the middle of his chemotherapy cycle and all of his hair had fallen out. Even though he wore a baseball cap, people stared at him constantly. The following dialogue took place during the walk:

Patient: I hate when people stare at me. It makes me feel upset and angry.
Therapist: Why do you think they stare at you?
Patient: Because my head has no hair.
Therapist: Do you think your hair will grow back?
Patient: The doctor said it would.
Therapist: Perhaps we can come up with something for you to say to yourself that can make you feel better when you think that people are staring at you.
Patient: Like what?
Therapist: What about "My hair will grow back soon. The medicine is helping my body to get strong again. They would also look funny with no hair. I can handle them staring at me. I'm not going to let them get me upset." Do you like any of these ideas?
Patient: Yes (laughing), I'm not going to let them make me so angry.
Therapist: So what could you think next time you think someone is staring at you?
Patient: I'll say, "They would look funny too with no hair but my hair will grow back so I can handle them staring."

The above technique is the direct method of teaching children to use coping self-statements. When using this method, the therapist suggests several coping self-statements and then asks the child if he or she would like to try them. The therapist then encourages the child to repeat the coping self-statements and reinforces the child for using them.

The Stuffed-animal Technique. An effective cognitive-restructuring method for children involves the use of stuffed animals. This technique may be especially useful for children ages 4 to 8 years old. We have found that this age group of children responds particularly well to the use of the stuffed animals. When using this technique, the therapist tells the child that one animal is sick and the other one is a best friend. The therapist and the child pretend that the best friend stuffed animal is giving advice to the sick stuffed animal. The child, with the help of the therapist, can then begin to write a list of coping self-statements generated by the advice of the sick stuffed animal. This technique enables the therapist to teach the child how to generate coping self-statements that the child can use for him or herself.

Robert, a 6-year-old boy, was brought to therapy to help him cope with his treatment for leukemia. His parents reported that he had temper tantrums and cried whenever he had to undergo chemotherapy. Several sessions were spent using the stuffed-animal technique. Whenever Robert produced a coping self-statement, the therapist gave him a Ninja Turtle sticker. He made believe that a teddy bear was giving a stuffed rabbit advice on how to get through chemotherapy sessions. Robert was able to come up with the following coping self-statements: "You're a big boy and can handle this. You'll feel strong again. The medicine will make you healthy. The hospital is a place where you get better. When you're better, you won't have to be here so much." Robert was encouraged to use the coping self-statements during the chemotherapy and received small toys as rewards from his parents after being cooperative with medical staff. Robert's parents reported that he was less resistant and cooperated with the medical staff during chemotherapy. The tantrums stopped and he exhibited less distress during his chemotherapy.

The Blackboard Technique. A technique that works well with older children (10 years and older) is a variation of the two-column method. Here, instead of using paper, a large blackboard is used with a line drawn down the middle. Both patient and therapist work together to come up with a list of coping self-statements to replace self-defeating negative thoughts. Once the list is generated, the therapist can usually persuade the child to copy the list and take it home to practice. Children tend to comply easily with this request and parents usually report that the list is tacked up on a bedroom wall where the child can look at it frequently.

Once children learn the fundamentals of developing coping self-statements, the therapist can then begin to help the child apply them in stressful situations. Children are usually willing to follow the therapist's instructions. Positive reinforcement can be used to encourage compliance. Candy, small toys, or stickers can be given as rewards to children whenever they apply the coping self-statements in stressful situations. In addition, relaxation and imagery techniques can also be employed for helping children cope with difficult situations.

Relaxation Training With Children

Children tend to be fearful about learning and using relaxation techniques unless the procedures are simplified and shortened. Children want and will use techniques that they can learn quickly and easily. Elliott and Ozolins (1983) developed a simple relaxation procedure for children. They taught children to take deep breaths and then to make a hissing sound such as "s-s-s-s-s," as they exhale. They also taught children to use coping statements, such as, "I know I can do it," along with the breathing exercises.

Chapter 3 describes the use of relaxation procedures for adults. We have modified these techniques for use with children. Because of the limited attention span of most children, the techniques have been shortened. The therapist needs to pay particular attention to the child's level of concentration. If the child appears bored or uninterested, the therapist needs to remain patient and guide the child slowly through the process. As with adults, the room should be quiet and the light in the room should be dim. The therapist can then use the same guidelines outlined in chapter 3, except in a more simplified manner.

Relaxation training is presented to children as a way of reducing pain and fear. Children are given simple instructions to take deep breaths and to then pretend that they are a loose and limp rag doll. Children practice relaxation during therapy sessions and are instructed to practice techniques at home as well. The therapist can teach the relaxation techniques to the parents so that they can practice with their child.

Terri, a 9-year-old girl with leukemia, hated going to the hospital for treatment. She would often have a temper tantrum and cry uncontrollably. Her parents became frustrated and did not know how to handle the situation. Terri was taught a very simple breathing exercise. She was told to take a deep breath, feel the breath in her tummy, and then slowly let it out. She also used coping self-statements along with the relaxation. She said to herself, "I can handle this," and imagined that her body was just like one of her rag dolls. She practiced this technique repeatedly until she mastered it. Her parents reported that this technique helped to calm her down when she became anxious and thus enabled her hospital treatments to continue as scheduled.

There are several studies in which relaxation training or hypnotic procedures similar to relaxation (see chapter 4) were employed for reducing distress from chemotherapy (Cotanch et al., 1985; Dolgin, Katz, McGinty, & Siegel, 1985; LaBaw et al., 1975; LeBaron & Zeltzer, 1984; Zeltzer et al., 1983, 1984). Relaxation procedures are also used as a part of various multicomponent programs developed for helping children cope with chemotherapy, bone marrow aspirations (BMAs), lumbar punctures, venopunctures, finger sticks, and other invasive medical procedures. These will be described later in the chapter.

Positive Reinforcement

The use of positive reinforcement is a very powerful technique that often helps children deal more successfully with painful medical procedures. Parents are often involved in this technique because they are the primary persons involved in transporting the child to the doctor's office or hospital for these invasive medical procedures. Parents can be taught to use positive reinforcement in several ways. The child can earn points or gold stars for each successful visit to the doctor. The stars or points can be exchanged at some point for tangible rewards, such as toys, trips to the movies or zoo, or even a special meal in a restaurant if the child feels up to it. The parents are also instructed to use verbal praise as an additional reinforcer. The therapist clarifies for the parents exactly what behaviors are to be reinforced. The children can either be rewarded for cooperation with the medical staff or be reinforced for utilizing their coping techniques, such as using relaxation and coping self-statements. In addition, the children can be taught to use covert reinforcement which involves imagining receiving a reward such as going to the toy store. The child might visualize receiving or playing with the reward and/or use self-statements, such as, "I can handle this, it won't be long before I'm finished at the doctor's office and will be on my way to the toy store." The therapist can also use small toys as rewards when the child has successfully employed cognitive-behavioral techniques. Some examples of rewards are small, inexpensive stuffed animals or inexpensive little people toys such as G.I. Joe or Teenage Mutant Ninja Turtles. As described in chapter 2, the Jay et al. (1985, 1987) program used small trophies as a reward for children who cooperated during medical procedures such as BMAs and spinal taps.

The parents are taught basic behavioral principles of identifying a target response (how the parent would like the child to behave), shaping the response (i.e., successive approximations) and then giving a positive reinforcement. One family rewarded their 8-year-old child with a weekend trip to a hotel for cooperation with each chemotherapy cycle (approximately four treatments). The child loved to go to hotels and have room service. In addition, he received small toys for applying his coping tools (coping self-statements and relaxation) during each chemotherapy treatment. Parents need guidance in applying behavioral principles. Usually, they apply these principles and report that they are effective in helping the children cope and comply with the medical procedures. The parents give the therapist a verbal report that helps the therapist in planning future behavioral strategies with the child and the family.

Reinforcement From Others

It is essential that significant others in the child's environment be involved in the treatment process. The significant others include the immediate family, siblings, relatives, friends, hospital staff, and attending physicians. These individuals can be taught the cognitive-behavioral coping techniques and how to use verbal reinforcement. These significant others not only help the child to cope more effectively but also help the parents to cope with the situation. The therapist plays the role of educator in this process. More will be said about this in the family chapter.

Imagery Techniques

Imagery training has been a useful cognitive-behavioral strategy that therapists have utilized with adults for any number of different situations. Imagery can also be used successfully with children. We have used imagery techniques with children in order to help them cope more effectively with their thoughts and feelings concerning their medical treatment procedures.

Emotive Imagery. A technique similar to emotive imagery (Lazarus & Abramovitz, 1962) that is especially effective with children ages 5 to 9 involves the use of superheroes and fantasy scenarios. The purpose of emotive imagery is to reduce anxiety and phobic avoidance. In its application to children with cancer, emotive imagery can be used to help them cope with invasive medical procedures. By becoming absorbed in the fantasy, the child is distracted, which reduces pain and anxiety. In addition, the fantasy can be constructed in such a manner that the meaning of the experience is altered so as to make it less threatening. For example, the child and the therapist create a scenario where the child has been asked by a superhero such as Batman to help all the other boys and girls in the world by taking an experimental serum. The superhero and the child are both aware that the serum can cause side effects much like the ones the child is experiencing from chemotherapy. However, because the child has been asked by the superhero to help, the child fantasizes, "I can be brave, I can handle this, and this will make the superhero (Batman) so proud of me. It will also help all the other sick boys and girls." The therapist encourages the child to participate as much as possible in constructing the story and praises the child whenever he or she comes up with a coping self-statement that can be combined with the imagery. This technique can be done while the child is in a relaxed or hypnotic state, or be used by itself. The therapist describes the story to the child, elaborating as much as possible on details relevant to the child's specific situation. The procedure can be recorded on a cassette tape which the child can take to the chemotherapy or radiation therapy treatments.

Distraction

As described in the previous chapter on pain control, distraction has been used by adults and children as a coping technique. As discussed in the chapter on stress management, relaxation training and hypnosis were found to help adult patients cope more effectively with chemotherapy. These techniques may be effective because of the process of distraction (Redd et al., 1987). Redd et al. (1987) used video-game playing as a way of distracting children undergoing chemotherapy from their nausea. They found that patients who used the video game for cognitive-attentional distraction experienced significantly less nausea than control subjects who received no treatment. Kolko and Rickard-Figueroa (1985) also found that engaging in video-game playing reduced distress in children undergoing chemotherapy.

Multicomponent Programs

As discussed earlier, although anxiety is a predominant emotion in children with cancer, they frequently have trouble expressing these feelings and instead tend to engage in acting-out behavior. Children become especially anxious just prior to medical procedures such as chemotherapy, radiation therapy, bone marrow aspirations, lumbar punctures, and blood tests. They often begin to cry, have temper tantrums, become nauseous, and sometimes vomit in anticipation of visits to the doctor for a treatment. Several studies have suggested that the combination of various cognitive-behavioral procedures like modeling, behavioral rehearsal, imagery, distraction, coping self-statements, and positive reinforcement significantly reduce children's distress in response to dental and surgical procedures (Melamed & Siegel, 1975; Nocella & Kaplan, 1982; Peterson & Shigetomi, 1981; Siegel & Peterson, 1980).

Several studies have demonstrated that multicomponent programs, based on stress-inoculation training, are effective in reducing distress in children with cancer undergoing BMAs (Jay et al., 1987, 1985) and in reducing distress during chemotherapy (Dahlquist et al., 1985). Details of the Jay et al. (1985, 1987) programs were described in the previous chapter on pain control. In the Dahlquist et al. program, muscle relaxation, breathing techniques, pleasant imagery, and positive self-statements were employed in helping children cope with chemotherapy.

Programs for Enhancing Life

The most striking aspect of cancer is the life-threatening nature of the disease. Van Dongen-Melman and Sanders-Woudstra (1986) report that children with cancer experience significant anxiety. Children become aware that the illness may lead to death. This awareness may not be overtly expressed. However, the children seem to develop "death anxiety." Spincetta and Maloney (1975) note that children with cancer experience more anxiety as the disease progresses. It appears that even though the child may be making progress with remission and treatment, a certain amount of uncertainty and fear of relapse is always present.

As described previously in the depression chapter, Cousins (1989), Le Shan (1977), Siegel (1986), Spiegel, Bloom, Kraemer, and Gottheil (1989) and Simonton et al. (1978) have developed programs for helping patients prolong life. The Simonton program entails the use of relaxation techniques and healing imagery. We have modified this approach for treatment of children with cancer. Our modification involves the use of the video game called Pac-Man. This is a game where Pac-Man (a good character) chases ghost-like creatures around a video screen and eventually eats them up. The goal is to eat up as many ghosts as you possibly can. The child can imagine that the ghosts are the cancer cells and that Pac-Man is an antibody. While playing the game, the child can imagine that Pac-Man is eating up all the cancer cells. Then, as a method for coping with chemotherapy, the child can fantasize that the chemotherapy consists of thousands of Pac-Men eating up the cancer cells. During the game, some children use coping self-statements, such as, "I'm going to get well, my medicine is going to make me healthy, I'm going to get rid of those cancer cells." This technique reduces feelings of anxiety as well as helplessness and hopelessness, and children enjoy participating in their treatment.

SUMMARY

In this chapter we have discussed how traditional play-therapy techniques can be integrated with cognitive-behavior therapy techniques in treating children with cancer. Cognitive-behavior therapy techniques that have been employed with adults need to be modified and simplified in order to be applicable with children. In order to find methods that will be effective with a particular child, the therapist needs to be creative and willing to experiment. Some mention has been made of the need to involve parents and significant others. The next chapter will deal with the effects of the illness on the family and some of the ways in which the family members may learn to better manage their feelings surrounding the illness.

Chapter 6
Working With the Family

A very important part of the treatment of a cancer patient involves the family members. When a family is directly involved in the treatment of a cancer patient they have a greater sense of control and also an opportunity to prepare themselves and the patient appropriately for each stage of the disease (Lansdown & Goldman, 1988). All family members are encouraged to participate in the treatment of the cancer patient. Family members assist the therapist by applying cognitive-behavioral principles and interventions in the home environment. They provide additional support, understanding, coaching, and back-up at home.

As our techniques for helping patients have been developed through the years, we have come to recognize how vital the role of the family is to the well-being of the cancer patient. When we first began to treat cancer patients with cognitive-behavior therapy techniques, we noticed that the families often exhibited a sense of helplessness. They would drive the patient to the office, wait outside in the waiting room, look encouraging, smile whenever possible, then take the patient home and repeat the cycle weekly. The initial reactions of the family have been studied in the literature. Anxiety, grief, anger, hostility, guilt, and disbelief are among the responses most often observed in families (Bozeman et al., 1955; Chodoff, Friedman & Hamburg, 1964; Lascari & Stehbens, 1973; Natterson & Knudson, 1960). In addition, the initial response of family members often includes the expectation that death is near. This thought, coupled with the above-mentioned emotions, often has a paralyzing effect on the family.

RATIONALE FOR FAMILY COUNSELING

Helplessness and loss of control are two feelings that patients and families often experience. The sense of helplessness experienced by indi-

90

vidual family members can have a very deleterious effect on the cancer patient. For example, stress and feelings of helplessness can build up and contribute to family arguments, especially between the parents. The child with cancer may then feel guilty and responsible for causing the parents to fight. Distress over the situation can affect various family members. Family members may become depressed to the point where they have difficulty functioning. Others may develop symptoms such as tension and migraine headaches, ulcers, or other stress-related disorders.

In addition, family members who feel helpless concerning the patient's illness may inadvertently convey these negative feelings to the patient. The patient in turn develops a sense of helplessness.

Although cognitive-behavior therapy is usually thought of as a treatment for individual patients, it can be viewed in the context of a larger system, that being the family. Teichman (1984) believes that integrating the family into cognitive-behavioral treatment helps build a meaningful frame of reference for explaining, diagnosing, and treating a wide range of problems of adjustment. Maladaptive feelings, such as helplessness and hopelessness, anger, guilt, and anxiety, are reduced by involving the family in the cancer patient's psychological treatment. The family begins to feel more in control when they too are taught what they can do to help.

Most family members are very receptive to having family sessions and they experience a sense of relief upon learning that they will be included in the cancer patient's therapy. For example, the parents of a little girl diagnosed with a malignant tumor came in to find out about psychotherapy for their child. The therapist explained the various techniques and concepts that could be used. They were also invited to attend some of the therapy sessions. At first they looked puzzled and then the father said, "You mean we get to help her in her treatment." "Yes," the therapist responded. "It's about time somebody let us do something to help," he replied.

MAJOR PSYCHOLOGICAL PROBLEMS CONFRONTING THE FAMILY OF THE CANCER PATIENT

The medical diagnosis of cancer causes a radical change in the normal day-to-day emotional functioning of both the patient and the patient's family. There is an upheaval of normal routine and an increase in the stress levels of the patient and family. If there were family problems prior to the onset of the illness, they are likely to be exacerbated after the diagnosis. One of the major problems facing the family is learning to cope with the emotions that may be evoked by the onset of cancer. Many patients and their families have difficulty adjusting to the diagnosis of cancer.

Greer (1988) developed the concept of "mental adjustment to cancer." "Mental adjustment" refers to the cognitive and behavioral responses of individuals to the diagnosis of cancer. Greer found that responses may be grouped in four broad categories: "stoic acceptance," a fatalistic outlook in which the diagnosis of cancer is just accepted; "denial," in which individuals avoid thinking about the cancer; "helplessness and hopelessness," in which individuals feel engulfed by the illness and have an impending sense of gloom; and "fighting spirit" in which an optimistic attitude and a desire to fight the cancer is adopted. Although Greer originally developed this classification to describe individuals' reactions to the diagnosis, we find it pertains to families as well.

Guilt and Anger

When a family finds out that one of its members has been diagnosed with cancer, common emotional reactions experienced by family members include guilt and anger. Guilt feelings may result from thinking of oneself as "bad" for having done something wrong, though the individual may not have actually done anything wrong. It may only be his or her belief or someone else's opinion. Some examples of guilt-producing thoughts include, "I shouldn't have hurt Phil's feelings," "I should have said I love you to Dad," "I should have done more for Mom." Family members who feel guilty may engage in overcompensation. For example, a parent might give a child with cancer more attention than the other children in the family. Overcompensation by a parent may cause resentment in siblings who may then act out their feelings in some manner. For example, another child in the family may begin to develop problems in school as a response to the overcompensation by the parents. As discussed in chapter 2, guilt is a form of depression. Family members may exhibit signs of depression such as missing work or withdrawing from social contacts. Methods for dealing with guilt will be discussed later in the chapter.

Anger may cause disruptions within the family structure. Anger may come from various sources. Other family members may resent the attention given to the cancer patient. The anger may be acted out in the form of hostility or be expressed passive-aggressively. When expressed passive-aggressively, a family member may neglect some of his or her responsibilities within the family, such as forgetting to pick something up at a store. In extreme situations, hostility may result in arguments or even physical acting out, such as hitting another family member. Cognitive-behavioral strategies for anger control will be discussed later in the chapter. In addition, we have found that maintaining a normal routine tends to prevent angry feelings from getting out of control. Within the context of a normal routine, we encourage the family to distribute attention as evenly as possible among the siblings and other family members. When everyone in the family feels that they are actually involved in the patient's treatment, it helps to minimize anger. Maintaining a normal routine will be discussed in greater depth later in the chapter.

Stress and Anxiety

After the diagnosis of cancer, the family's life and lifestyle become radically changed. In addition to coping with the stresses of their everyday routine, they must learn to cope with the onset of new stresses. Chesler and Barbarin (1987) describe the five different types of stresses caused by the onset of the illness: intellectual stress, created by the massive amount of technical information about the disease and its treatment that the family members will need to learn; instrumental stress, created by the establishment of new daily tasks involved in maintaining a home, family, and work life in the midst of the medical problems; interpersonal stress, created by the escalating needs of all family members and the changing sets of relations with old and new friends and with health service providers; emotional stress, created by the psychological consequences of fear, distress, and loss of sleep and energy; and existential stress, created by confusion about the meaning and order of life which has been upset by the onset of the illness.

The family can learn techniques to help them manage the above-mentioned stresses and anxieties. Stress management was described in detail in chapter 3. When applied to family treatment, the same methods are used, only in a group setting. Families are taught techniques such as relaxation and cognitive restructuring as a group. They can discuss common stressors, or the focus can be on an individual. If necessary, the therapist can also meet with family members on an individual basis.

BASIC PRINCIPLES IN COGNITIVE-BEHAVIOR FAMILY THERAPY

We have developed some basic principles in working with families using cognitive-behavior therapy. The basic principles that are utilized are designed to build a supportive network involving the patient, the family, the extended family, significant others in the patient's life, and the therapist. The major goals of the therapy are to educate the network members to the basic techniques of cognitive-behavior therapy and to try to maintain as normal a routine as possible during the medical treatment.

Extended Family Involvement

In addition to primary family involvement, it is strongly suggested that the family enlist the help of extended family members. Aunts, uncles, grandparents, and cousins can all be used to help both the patient and the family. They can help in a supportive role, such as babysitting other children when the parents have to stay in the hospital with their child with cancer. They can visit hospitalized family members, help out with driving the patient to his or her medical treatments, pick up medications from drugstores when needed, and make themselves generally available to help the immediate family.

The Use of Significant Others

Besides involving extended family members, the immediate family can utilize the help of close friends, neighbors, schoolmates, and other families of cancer patients. We have found that the larger the support system the more it can help the family to cope with the crisis at hand. Chesler and Barbarin (1987) strongly suggest that families not feel that they are going through the crisis alone. It is important for the immediate family to seek many sources of help and support and to learn that the people around them are concerned and care about them. Lansdown and Goldman (1988), in discussing the stress on the family, also recommend that the family involve as many significant others as they can in order to help build a supportive, caring network. It is also recommended that the hospital team help the family to find other appropriate support networks, such as the Candlelighters or the Make-A-Wish Foundation, to help them cope with the illness. More will be discussed about supportive networks later on in the chapter.

The Role of the Therapist

The therapist's role during initial sessions with a family is to determine and assess each individual family member's cognitive, emotional, and behavioral reactions to the diagnosis of cancer. Many family members are so shocked and upset about the diagnosis that they become paralyzed with respect to normal functioning. This may prevent them from the important process of information gathering. One of the major roles of the therapist is to advise the family about how and where to get information about the illness. Families educated about the illness can offer more support and understanding to the cancer patient during the various treatment phases.

Another role of the therapist is to help the family cope rationally and effectively with the material they have gathered concerning the illness. When families gather information about the particular type of cancer they are dealing with, they tend to dwell on the disastrous experiences that they have heard about. The therapist can diffuse the anxiety elicited by these "horror" stories by pointing out that each case is unique. Although it may be a similar cancer, everyone reacts differently and it is difficult to draw parallels from one case to another. Clarification by the oncologist and the therapist helps a family to rationally understand their specific problem and the way it affects their family member.

The therapist can also play an important role when it comes to the hospitalization of the cancer patient. During initial family sessions, it is important for the therapist to prepare the family for the possibility of hospitalization. The therapist can teach the family that hospitalization does not necessarily mean a disastrous outcome. The therapist helps the family to cope with the stress involved in hospitalization and helps them make decisions concerning the family member's treatment.

The therapist also has the task of understanding the dynamics, background, and communication style of the family. The therapist's role is to design a treatment program consistent with the family's needs and idiosyncratic structure (Minuchin, 1974; Teichman, 1984; Welch-McCaffrey, 1983).

Maintaining a Normal Routine

We have found that, as a working principle, when and wherever possible, it is best to encourage families to live their lives as normally as possible in spite of the illness. Every member of the family is encouraged to go about their own particular activities as normally as possible. Obviously this precludes any emergency or unexpected event such as a hospitalization. For example, several years ago a patient and his family had an opportunity to take a trip to California. The family's immediate response was to decline the trip. They felt that a trip might be too taxing on the patient. The patient wanted very much to go, especially to see Disneyland. Problem solving was used to help them make a decision. The therapist helped them to weigh the pros and cons of such a trip with regards to how it might affect the patient and the family. As part of the problem solving, the therapist asked the family if they would go had the patient never been diagnosed with cancer. The family responded that there would be no question about going on the trip. The therapist educated the family about the importance of maintaining a normal routine. Further problem solving focused on possible medical situations and other problems that could arise. The therapist guided the family in arriving at rational approaches for dealing with potential problems that might occur, such as finding an attending physician, connecting with a hospital in California, communicating with their oncologist back in New York, and dealing with the need for any possible medications. After lengthy discussions of these issues, the family decided that if the oncologist gave his permission to go, then the family would go. Because the patient's medical treatment was proceeding without any problems, the family went on the trip, which had a positive effect on the patient. During a session after the trip, the father reiterated how important it was for them to go away and act as a normal family.

Generally, patients tend to respond better psychologically when they feel that their lifestyle is as normal as possible. The motivation for normalcy can be a powerful tool in teaching coping skills and problem solving to the family. As a further example of this principle, one teenager with bone cancer insisted on being in school whenever possible. She intended to graduate with her class and continue on to college. She and her family agreed on this and tried very hard to maintain as normal a routine as possible. The teenager felt that this helped her maintain a sense of control over at least some aspects of her life.

BASIC TECHNIQUES

Families can benefit from learning cognitive-behavior therapy techniques. The goal in teaching cognitive-behavior therapy to the family is twofold. First, the techniques can be used by family members to cope with their own feelings. Second, family members understand what the patient needs to do to cope with his or her feelings. These techniques can be taught to the entire family during sessions or the therapist has the option of working with individual family members during the privacy of individual sessions. Families tend to respond very positively to learning these techniques. One family reported that they felt more comfortable dealing with their daughter's oncologist in terms of asking him questions as a result of learning stress-management techniques and assertiveness skills. Families are taught cognitive restructuring, problem solving, relaxation training, assertiveness training, and how to validate feelings.

Assertiveness Training

Assertiveness is beyond the scope of this book. The reader is referred to other sources such as Fensterheim and Baer (1975) and Lange and Jakubowski (1976). However, here are several guidelines for teaching assertiveness:

1. When expressing feelings, use "I" statements. For example, "I feel annoyed."
2. Do not blame the other person or make global evaluations. Comment on specific behaviors. For example, "I feel annoyed when you come home late" instead of "You're always late."
3. Tell the person what you woul.' like him or her to do. Make a suggestion. For example, "If you are going to be late, I would like you to call me."
4. Try to state your feelings calmly. When expressing anger, avoid yelling or name calling.

The therapist teaches the family how to validate feelings by incorporating the following guidelines:

1. Do not interrupt the other person while he or she is speaking.
2. Acknowledge the other person's feelings by using active listening. Paraphrase your understanding of what the other person is saying and feeling. Keep in mind that acknowledgment is not equated with agreement.
3. Check to make sure that you have understood the other person correctly before expressing your viewpoint. Only the other person can determine whether he or she has been understood.

The therapist teaches the family how to recognize, express, and validate feelings such as anger, guilt, anxiety, and depression. The therapist explains that it is unhealthy to suppress feelings. The therapist points out that suppressed feelings can intensify stress and anger and may lead to stress-related symptoms or maladaptive behavior such as excessive alcohol consumption. Family members are taught to accept themselves with whatever feelings they experience. They are taught that feelings are neither right nor wrong, and it is desirable to express them in an assertive, not hostile, manner. When anger takes the form of hostility, or rage, it can have a disruptive effect on the family. Therefore, another therapeutic approach involves teaching family members to reduce the intensity of their emotions. Anger reduction will be discussed later in the chapter.

Cognitive Restructuring

Ellis (1962), Beck (1976), and Meichenbaum (1977) describe cognitive restructuring as a means of modifying the patient's irrational beliefs, self-defeating thoughts, faulty premises and erroneous assumptions. The therapist helps the family to identify their self-defeating and irrational thoughts and teaches them how to think more rationally. Family members can be taught how to use coping self-statements as described in previous chapters.

The following example demonstrates how cognitive restructuring can be taught to an entire family. An 8-year-old boy, receiving chemotherapy, was hospitalized for an infection. The infection was caused by the insertion of a Broviac tube (a device used to help deliver chemotherapy to children instead of using veins which may collapse and cause the child discomfort). This procedure was relatively minor and went very well except for the onset of the infection. The infection caused a high fever which necessitated the ensuing hospitalization. The family became very upset and concerned. However, during a family counseling session, the therapist and family discussed how to handle the crisis. The therapist asked them to identify their anxiety-producing thoughts. Various family members had thoughts such as, "This is probably the beginning of the end," "Joey will never recover," and "Hospitalization during treatment means certain death." The therapist pointed out how they were jumping to conclusions and suggested alternative ways of viewing the situation, such as, "We need to learn all the details of the hospitalization before reaching a conclusion," "Patients do become hospitalized during treatment," "Infections during Broviac surgery are common," and "Hospitalization doesn't necessarily mean death." The therapist also taught them how to use coping self-statements for reducing anxiety, such as, "Calm down, learn the facts," "Keep things in perspective and deal with the situation," "Infections are common in children." By learning these techniques, the family was able to cope successfully with the hospitalization and continued to provide support for the patient.

A second example of the value of cognitive restructuring occurred during a hospital visit. The therapist (D.M.R.) had the opportunity to observe a particular situation and play an intervening role that was helpful to a family member. The cancer patient was readmitted to the hospital because of stomach pains. The patient was connected to intravenous tubes and appeared in pain. A nurse had to rub the patient down with lotion in order to prevent bedsores. The patient's older brother became very upset at the way the nurse was handling his brother. The nurse was working very carefully but the patient was in a lot of pain. The patient's brother began to interfere and get in the way of the nurse. The therapist approached the brother and began to talk with him about the situation:

Therapist: What are you feeling?
Patient: I'm upset.
Therapist: What are you thinking about?
Patient: She's hurting my brother. He's in enough pain. She should be more considerate and caring. She should know he's in pain.

Therapist: Remember back to our family sessions. I know you're upset but think the situation through. Is the nurse hurting your brother on purpose? Do you think she's doing the best she can under the circumstances?

Patient: No, not on purpose. I realize she's doing the best she can and she's really trying to help him.

Therapist: How do you feel now?

Patient: A little calmer and certainly more in control.

Therapist: Good! Let's go back inside.

The brother regained his composure and returned to the room much less upset.

Problem Solving

We have found it very useful to teach problem-solving techniques to families of cancer patients. Goldfried and Davison (1976) define problem solving as a technique that provides a variety of potentially effective responses to the problem situation and increases the likelihood of selecting the most effective response from various alternatives. Problem-solving skills help families to cope more effectively with the challenges presented to them by the nature of the illness.

Families are taught the following steps in problem solving:

1.   define the problem
2.   list alternative ways of coping with the problem
3.   evaluate the various alternatives, think of the advantages and disadvantages of each alternative
4.   select the alternative or set of alternatives with the most advantages and the least disadvantages
5.   implement and evaluate the effectiveness of the alternative(s) and if the outcome is unsuccessful, go back to the first step and repeat the process

Families that learn the technique of problem solving seem to function at higher levels than families that do not have this skill when faced with a crisis. An example of problem solving was described earlier with regard to a family trying to decide whether or not to go on their trip to California.

Another example of problem solving involved a family that was having some problems dealing with an oncologist. The problem involved their difficulty in obtaining information from the oncologist. The family defined the problem as their feeling intimidated by the oncologist and that they were fearful of asking him any questions because of his evasive answers. The therapist then asked them to generate a list of alternative ways of coping with the doctor. The list included alternatives such as switching to another oncologist, being more assertive with the present oncologist, and the therapist talking to the oncologist. The family decided that the most rational, logical thing to do was to be more assertive and confront the doctor. They felt he was a good oncologist and decided against switching doctors. The therapist then taught them some assertive skills. Through modeling and role play, the therapist showed the parents how to confront the oncologist without sounding hostile. Although the oncologist was not particularly receptive, the parents nevertheless felt more in control in their dealings with him.

Information Gathering

Information gathering is an important skill for families. The therapist encourages the family to use all resources that may be available. Personal computers can be used for this purpose. One father of a child diagnosed with a malignant brain tumor used his personal computer to access many different data bases to gather medical information about cases similar to his daughter's.

The therapist can also help educate the family about the availability of support groups and self-help literature. Support groups are important because the members of these groups have gone through, or are going through, similar experiences. Support groups offer emotional reassurance, as well as opportunities to network and learn more about additional resources.

One of the major organizations that also serves as a support group is the American Cancer Society (ACS). The ACS usually holds weekly or monthly support-group meetings. Outside sponsors, doctors, or therapists are often invited to come to the meetings and speak on a topic of interest. Presentations are followed by a social hour providing the participants a chance to get to know one another. The ACS will also provide referrals to other organizations that have been formed to help cancer patients and their families. One such organization is the Make-A-Wish Foundation. This particular group will grant special wishes to children, such as an all-expenses-paid trip to Disneyworld or an afternoon lunch with a famous star. Another organization is the Candlelighter's Organization, a support group for the parents of children with life-threatening illnesses. They provide Christmas parties, picnics, and information resources for the family. Another organization is the Brain Tumor Foundation. This group is dedicated to raising money for research on brain tumors. Therapists can learn about the availability of additional groups through the ACS.

It is recommended that the therapist familiarize him or herself with the self-help literature. The therapist may find it helpful to recommend several self-help books to the family of cancer patients. Some of these books include *I Want to Grow Hair, I Want to Grow Up, I Want to Go to Boise: Children Surviving Cancer* (Bombeck, 1989), *A Comprehensive Guide for Cancer Patients and Families* (Rosenbaum & Rosenbaum, 1980) and *A New Guide to Rational Living* (Ellis & Harper, 1975). We have found that self-help books provide additional support for the family and reinforce the concepts and techniques taught to them during family-therapy sessions.

APPLICATIONS

Cognitive-behavior therapy techniques can be applied to a number of different problems experienced by families coping with cancer. We will now deal specifically with overcoming guilt, anger control, recurrence of the illness, and grief counseling.

Overcoming Guilt

Guilt was discussed in chapter 2 on depression. As mentioned in that chapter, guilt stems from self-condemnation. When individuals feel guilt, it is because they believe they are worthless or no good because of some presumed wrongdoing. They may not have done anything wrong. The family members of cancer patients often jump to conclusions about how they "wronged" the patient. For example, the statement, "I shouldn't have made Bobbie angry at me" might be the automatic response of a sibling. The therapist teaches the family members that guilt is often experienced when one learns that a loved one has cancer. The therapist helps the family members to question their automatic assumptions about whether or not they actually did anything wrong. They are also taught to accept themselves even if they made mistakes or did do something wrong. For example, a 12-year-old boy felt guilty because he believed fighting with his 9-year-old brother contributed to the cancer. The therapist explained that fighting between brothers is normal and does not cause cancer. The 12-year-old also felt guilty for having hidden some of his brother's favorite toys. The therapist pointed out that although it was wrong to hide the toys, brothers often do that to one another and there was nothing that he did that caused the illness.

Anger Control

Typically, cancer patients and family members experience anger from the moment the diagnosis is given. Family members are often angry at anyone and everyone. Their thoughts are punctuated with "why us?" and "this shouldn't have happened to us." The therapist explains that no one can predict cancer and that most people in their situation feel the same, at least initially. The therapist validates their feelings, but explains how one can cope with anger. The therapist points out that anger may interfere with the ability to problem solve and be assertive. Anger may lead to hostility and impulsiveness. The therapist teaches the family how persistent rumination of angry thoughts causes excessive anger. The therapist can utilize stress-inoculation training (Novaco, 1975) for anger control. Several steps are involved in stress-inoculation training. Initially, families are taught relaxation and assertiveness. They are also taught how to rationally reevaluate their thoughts and how to develop coping self-statements for controlling anger. Then, they mentally rehearse how they could apply these skills. While in a relaxed state, they imagine coping with frustrations and provocations.

Stress-inoculation training was used with the father of a 5-year-old who had leukemia. After the diagnosis, he became extremely angry, to the point that it was affecting his relationships with fellow workers. He became impatient and hypercritical with subordinates, and got into arguments with them. His angry thoughts about his coworkers included, "They should know what I'm going through, they shouldn't bother me with petty details, they should try harder because of what I'm going through." Cognitive restructuring was employed and the following coping self-statements were developed: "This is my problem, they had nothing to do with it, some people have been sympathetic, but not everyone has to be, it's unrealistic to expect them to work harder because of my problem."

The father was taught relaxation. While in a relaxed state, he practiced the coping self-statements while imagining himself coping with situations such as coworkers making mistakes, asking him about details, and missing deadlines.

Coping With Recurrences

Unfortunately, we have treated cases where there have been recurrences of the cancer. After a recurrence, families enter the therapy room with an attitude and feeling of hopelessness. They feel beaten by the illness. If the family continues to respond with hopelessness it may affect the cancer patient's emotional and physical health.

The therapist has the difficult task of helping the family members cope with the recurrence. The role of the therapist is to console the family and help them continue to remain calm. The therapist provides the family with more rational ways of viewing the situation. For example, the wife of a cancer patient came into a family session quite upset. Her husband was just diagnosed with a recurrence of his cancer. She was convinced that his death was imminent and that nothing could be done. The therapist consoled her and began to help her to reevaluate her belief that the situation was hopeless. It was pointed out that 3 years ago, when he was originally diagnosed, his situation was serious. However, 3 years had passed and her husband had done well with his chemotherapy. He had succeeded at achieving several significant goals. The therapist asked her if the doctor had mentioned anything about an amount of time that her husband had left to live. The wife replied, "No!" "Then why are you giving up?" asked the therapist. The wife just shrugged her shoulders and said, "I don't know."

The therapist taught her to use cognitive restructuring and coping self-statements. He explained that many people catastrophize and assume the worst whenever there is a recurrence of the cancer. He further explained that catastrophizing only makes things worse by leading to feelings of helplessness and hopelessness. The therapist suggested several coping self-statements, such as, "Remain calm, learn all the facts," "When I'm calm I can help my husband in better ways," and "Stay focused and avoid jumping to conclusions — many patients who have had recurrences have survived and are still doing well." The woman used all of these suggestions successfully to cope with the situation.

Grief Counseling

We have experienced the loss of several patients. This is perhaps the most emotionally draining event that can happen to the family, and to the therapist. Kozier and Lea (1979) describe an approach for helping families with the five stages of grief initially described by Kübler-Ross (1969) for individuals. We have added cognitive-behavioral interventions to supplement their program.

Stage 1 is denial. During this stage the family exhibits nonacceptance of the event. They cannot believe that this has happened to them. The therapist helps the family by teaching them to confront the reality of the situation and to understand that death has occurred. They need help coming to terms with the reality of the death. The therapist can help in their adjustment by suggesting rational viewpoints such as the following, "Cancer is very unpredictable and no one really can predict what will happen or how it will affect any patient; the patient fought as hard as he could; the patient is no longer in any pain resulting from the illness." Stage 2 is anger. During this stage, the therapist validates and encourages the family members to express their feelings. However, if the anger is excessive or maladaptive, the therapist can introduce stress-inoculation training. Stage 3 is bargaining. Family members will typically say, "I'd do anything to change this." The therapist will need to listen attentively and be understanding and supportive. Stage 4 is depression. The family members begin to realize what they have lost. The therapist encourages the family members to express their feelings and not withdraw. The therapist also encourages the family to use interventions described in chapter 2 on depression. Stage 5 is acceptance of the death. This last stage takes considerable time and should not be hurried. We have found that it may take a year or more for someone to accept such a loss. Grief frequently reemerges even after considerable acceptance, such as when holidays, anniversaries, and birthdays occur.

SUMMARY

This chapter has demonstrated the importance of family involvement in the cancer patient's treatment. We have described methods for teaching families how to help the patient. We have also described techniques for helping family members cope with their own stress, depression, guilt, anger, and grief.

Chapter 7

Issues and Dilemmas of the Therapist — Directions for the Future

In the previous six chapters, we have sought to develop a comprehensive treatment approach for coping with cancer. In this chapter, we turn our attention to issues and dilemmas confronting the therapist working with cancer patients.

THERAPIST BURNOUT

Working in a clinical setting can be demanding and takes a great deal of expertise and personal involvement. We have found that working with cancer patients is especially difficult and stressful. Le Shan (1977) concluded on the basis of his work with cancer patients that it is too stressful for a therapist to work exclusively with this patient population.

Coping With Negative Emotions

There is a wide variety of emotions that can be aroused in the therapist working with cancer patients. Therapists need to be aware of emotions such as pity, anger, anxiety, and depression that interfere with objectivity and one's ability to deliver the best possible patient care.

Sympathy is easily aroused when working with seriously ill patients. Whereas empathy, concern, compassion, care, and sympathy are appropriate emotions for a therapist, pity is not. According to Hauck (1976), pity involves catastrophizing. As Hauck (1966) points out, if the therapist overtly or tacitly agrees with the patient's maladaptive beliefs and attitudes, therapeutic effectiveness will be compromised. Furthermore, if the therapist pities the patient with cancer, he or she can become depressed.

Therefore, it might be helpful for the therapist to recognize the signs or cues that reveal when he or she is becoming too personally involved. The therapist then needs to step back from the case by discussing his or her feelings with another therapist or engage in self-therapy. There are a number of self-help books based on cognitive-behavior therapy that can be used by the professional for self-therapy (e.g., Burns, 1984; Ellis & Harper, 1975; Hauck, 1976). These books are also excellent as bibliotherapy for patients. They can be used to teach patients the basics of cognitive-behavior therapy, as well as supplementing and reinforcing what takes place during therapy sessions. Of course, empathy for the patient is desirable and will often increase the efficacy of therapist involvement.

Pity is one type of depression. Another type of depression that can affect a therapist is the feeling of inadequacy. Depression can develop when the therapist blames him or herself for not helping or "curing" the patient. If the therapist has unrealistic expectations about what he or she can do to help the patient, when the patient dies or fails to respond to therapeutic interventions to relieve anxiety, depression, and pain, the therapist may think of him or herself as a failure. It is important that the therapist monitor these thoughts and dispute irrational thoughts, such as, "I should have been more helpful" or "I should have done more for this patient." Interestingly, these emotions are aroused partly because the therapist believes that he or she did not give the patient adequate treatment, when in fact, if asked, the patient may feel that the therapeutic interventions were quite helpful.

There are also treatment failures that occur because the patient is not ready or willing to be an active part of the therapy. Resistance to treatment will occur and the therapist can be aware of this so as not to be disappointed.

Further failures occur because some patients will not be successful with the treatment procedures outlined in this book. At those times that the treatment itself is a failure, the therapist can learn that he or she cannot expect success with every patient. Although this may sound simplistic, it is important to realize this fact so that the therapist does not think that he or she should be more successful with cancer patients than with the clinical population as a whole. In addition, if you are attempting these techniques for the first time or you do not have a large cancer population in your clinical practice, the limitations for success are greater due to inexperience.

Therefore, the therapist should not only be realistic about what can be accomplished, but should also recognize when he or she was in fact successful in helping a patient.

Coping With a Patient's Death

Mental health professionals do not typically work with illnesses that are life threatening, so therefore they often are ill-prepared to deal with the death of a patient. It is difficult to tell another professional how they are going to feel when they are confronted by this problem; although we can say that there may be an entire range of emotions that can and probably will be felt. Ellis and Harper (1975) point out that sadness is appropriate, whereas depression is not.

One of the ways therapists can prepare themselves for the death of their patients is to have an accurate and realistic picture of the patient's illness. The therapist is advised to be in contact with the patient's oncologist in order to determine the prognosis.

In addition, by working with the patient to accept death, the therapist can also learn to feel more comfortable about death. As previously mentioned in the book, positive thinking and "constructive denial," where the patient accepts the diagnosis but defies the prognosis, can be healthy for the patient. However, it is important for the therapist to also be able to acknowledge and discuss the patient's feelings about death, when it is suspected that the patient is experiencing anxiety or depression about the prospect of dying. If the patient resists exploring this topic, it is best for the therapist to acquiesce. One patient was very angry and terminated therapy when her previous therapist insisted that she had to talk about dying. The patient made it very clear to her new therapist that she wanted to "focus on living and not dying."

ADDITIONAL RESPONSIBILITIES

Treating cancer patients entails additional responsibilities that therapists do not usually encounter in clinical practice. Each additional responsibility confronts the therapist with difficult choices. The therapist may need to decide whether or not to visit patients in their homes or hospitals and go to funerals. Once, one of us was called upon to deliver a eulogy for a patient at his funeral. We will now discuss the issues surrounding some of these responsibilities.

Home Visitations

The office is the primary location for therapy. Unfortunately, when working with cancer patients this may not always be possible. Many times we have been confronted with patients who have told us that they were unable to continue treatment because they were home bound or hospitalized. We have discussed with these patients home visits and most of them have found this to be an acceptable alternative rather than terminating therapy.

Issues of billing for the extra time involved are up to the individual therapist, although if the demands on your schedule are not too severe in terms of distance to the patient's house, then billing for the same or a slightly larger fee is being sensitive to the patient's financial difficulties. There are other times when home visits can be used as a vehicle to say goodbye to the patient because he or she is too weak for actual therapy.

Hospital Visitations

There are times when the patient may have to be hospitalized while undergoing treatment. As with home visits, the therapist may want to continue treatment although the venue has changed. Some hospitals may not allow the therapist to be involved professionally so you may want to discuss with the patient that you are in the hospital as a visitor and not as the patient's therapist.

Telephone Calls

Many times during medical treatment, a patient may have to be hospitalized or have to stay home and miss a therapy appointment due to a medical complication. It is recommended that the therapist call and briefly talk with the patient. We have found that these telephone calls help to maintain the therapeutic relationship and can be helpful to the patient. Hospitals are lonely places and often visitors are scarce.

During the telephone calls, the therapist can offer continued encouragement and help to reinforce therapeutic suggestions that were developed during therapy sessions. It also portrays caring behavior to the patient and often this may help the patient to feel less anxious and tense.

Funerals

There are no rules or generally accepted guidelines concerning funeral attendance. The therapist can do as he or she feels comfortable doing, although an appearance at the funeral seems to provide the family with closure, especially if the family developed a close relationship with the therapist. Of course, the therapist cannot bill the family for attending the patient's funeral. In treating cancer patients, sometimes the therapist is called upon to go beyond the call of duty. Naturally, some therapists may not want to undertake these added responsibilities, and therapists do have the right to set limits.

ETHICAL DILEMMAS

Billing Problems

Many therapists have a great deal of difficulty when the patient has died and the final bill has to be presented to the family. They fear that they will be perceived as uncaring. A short period of mourning could be allowed before sending a bill, such as 2 weeks or as long as a month. After this time, the therapist should not feel uncomfortable about sending a bill for payment, as the services were rendered. Most families expect to receive these bills, as they are probably getting them from hospitals and oncologists as well as from the therapist. We feel that to ignore the final bill is to act as if you, the therapist, are responsible for the treatment outcome, which of course is not true.

Healing Imagery

Another issue faced by the clinician working with cancer patients is how to react to patients' requests for psychological techniques for prolonging life. The Simontons (Simonton et al., 1978) claim that healing imagery and meditation can be used by cancer patients to influence the course of their illness. Le Shan (1977) and Siegel (1986) report that they have helped patients induce a remission in their cancer as the result of lifestyle changes and positive thinking. Whether or not the clinician believes that this is possible, many patients strongly believe it is possible and request these types of interventions. How should the clinician respond? If we reject the patient's request and assert that it is a "crock," we very well might alienate and possibly demoralize the patient. On the other hand, we want to be responsible, ethical, and not make false claims or mislead the patient. Each therapist has to deal with this dilemma in a way that makes sense for him or her. Our approach has been to not promote these techniques. When our patients inquire about them, we honestly admit that we do not know whether or not they work. When asked for information, we provide it and educate our patients about these procedures and how they are used. We even help them to construct images about healing if this is what they request. Having patients imagine healing taking place seems to make them view the chemotherapy as a less negative experience. For example, one patient imagined the chemotherapy chemicals attacking the walls of the cancer cells, breaking down these walls, attacking the nuclei of the cancer cells, and destroying them. This imagery allowed the patient to feel he was actively participating in his treatment. With regards to children, if parents ask, "Can you use healing imagery with my child, I have heard it prolongs life," we take the same approach as previously described with adult patients.

AIDS and Cancer

It is beyond the scope of this book to discuss the psychological treatment of AIDS patients except for the obvious issue that many AIDS patients develop cancer as part of their disease. We find that there are similarities between working with AIDS patients and cancer patients. However, our experience with AIDS patients is limited. The reader is advised to consult Winiarski (1991) for information on AIDS-related psychotherapy.

FUTURE RESEARCH

Some research has already been conducted evaluating the efficacy of cognitive-behavioral methods for helping patients cope with invasive medical procedures. These studies have been discussed in previous chapters. We have also presented research on cognitive-behavioral treatments for pain, stress, and depression. Some research has also been conducted on programs that claim to prolong life and improve the quality of life. This area of research is in its infancy and is in need of further study.

We have described a number of techniques that we have found to be effective but have not been tested through research. It is our hope that this volume will stimulate research to further evaluate these methods. Working with children in particular has forced us to be innovative in developing new therapeutic methods. Research is needed to determine whether these methods are effective in the hands of other clinicians. We need to question whether a particular technique is effective because of its potency or if its effectiveness is attributable to other factors, such as the personality of the therapist. We encourage you to experiment with the techniques we have described and hope you will expand on our work.

References

Ament, P. (1982). Concepts in the use of hypnosis for pain relief in cancer. *Journal of Medicine, 13*, 233–240.

Araoz, D.L. (1983). Use of hypnotic techniques with oncology patients. *Journal of Psychosocial Oncology, 1*, 47–54.

Barber, J. (1978). Hypnosis as a psychological technique in the management of cancer pain. *Cancer Nursing, 1*, 361–363.

Barber, J., & Gitelson, J. (1980). Cancer pain: Psychological management using hypnosis. *Cancer: A Cancer Journal for Clinicians, 30*, 130–136.

Beck, A.T. (1976). *Cognitive therapy and emotional disorders.* New York: International Universities Press.

Beck, A.T., Hollon, S.D., Young, J.E., & Bedrosian, R.C. (1985). Treatment of depression with cognitive therapy and amitriptyline. *Archives of Psychiatry, 42*, 142–148.

Beck, A.T., Kovacs, M., & Weissman, A. (1975). Hopelessness and suicidal behavior: An overview. *Journal of the American Medical Association, 234*, 1146–1149.

Beck, A.T., Rush, A.J., Shaw, B.F., & Emery, G. (1979). *Cognitive therapy of depression.* New York: Guilford.

Beck, A.T., Weissman, A., Lester, D., & Trexler, L. (1974). The measurement of pessimism: The Hopelessness Scale. *Journal of Consulting and Clinical Psychology, 42*, 861–865.

Benson, H. (1975). *The relaxation response.* New York: Avon.

Blackburn, I.M., Bishop, S., Glen, A.I.M., Whalley, L.J., & Christie, J.E. (1981). The efficacy of cognitive therapy in depression: A treatment trial using cognitive therapy and pharmacotherapy, each alone and in combination. *British Journal of Psychiatry, 139*, 181–189.

Bombeck, E. (1989). *I want to grow hair, I want to grow up, I want to go to Boise: Children surviving cancer.* New York: Harper & Row.

Bonica, J.J. (1979). Importance of the problem. In J.J. Bonica & V. Ventafridda (Eds.), *Advances in pain research and therapy: Vol. 2.* New York: Raven Press.

Bonica, J.J. (1980). Cancer pain. In J.J. Bonica (Ed.), *Pain* (pp. 335–362). New York: Review Press.

Bozeman, M.F., Orbach, C.E., & Sutherland, A.M. (1955). Psychological impact of cancer and its treatment III. The adaptation of mothers to the threatened loss of their children through leukemia: Part I. *Cancer, 8*, 1–19.

Burish, T.G., & Carey, M.P. (1986). Conditioned aversive responses in cancer chemotherapy patients: Theoretical and developmental analysis. *Journal of Consulting and Clinical Psychology, 54,* 593–600.

Burish, T.G., Carey, M.P., Krozely, M.G., & Greco, F.A. (1987). Conditioned nausea and vomiting induced by cancer chemotherapy: Prevention through behavioral treatment. *Journal of Consulting and Clinical Psychology, 55,* 42–48.

Burish, T.G., & Lyles, J.N. (1979). Effectiveness of relaxation training in reducing the aversiveness of chemotherapy in the treatment of cancer. *Journal of Behavior Therapy and Experimental Psychiatry, 10,* 357–361.

Burish, T.G., & Lyles, J.N. (1981). Effectiveness of relaxation training in reducing adverse reactions to cancer chemotherapy. *Journal of Behavioral Medicine, 4,* 65–78.

Burns, D.D. (1984). *Feeling good: The new mood therapy.* New York: William Morrow.

Butler, B. (1954). The use of hypnosis in the care of the cancer patient. *Cancer, 7,* 1–14.

Cangello, V.M. (1961). The use of hypnotic suggestion for pain relief in malignant disease. *International Journal of Clinical and Experimental Hypnosis, 9,* 17–22.

Carey, M.P., & Burish, T.G. (1987). Providing relaxation training to cancer chemotherapy patients: A comparison of three methods. *Journal of Consulting and Clinical Psychology, 55,* 732–737.

Carey, M.P., & Burish, T.G. (1988). Etiology and treatment of the psychological side effects associated with cancer chemotherapy: A critical review and discussion. *Psychological Bulletin, 104,* 307–325.

Cassileth, B.R., Lusk, E.J., Miller, D.S., Brown, L.L., & Miller, C. (1985). Psychosocial correlates of survival in advanced malignant disease. *New England Journal of Medicine, 312,* 1551.

Chesler, M.A., & Barbarin, O.A. (1987). *Childhood cancer and the family.* New York: Brunner/Mazel.

Chodoff, P., Friedman, S.B., & Hamburg, D.A. (1964). Stress, defenses and coping behavior: Observations in parents of children with malignant disease. *American Journal of Psychiatry, 120,* 743–749.

Cleeland, C.S., & Tearnan, B.H. (1986). Behavioral control of cancer pain. In A.D. Holzman & D.C. Turk (Eds.), *Pain management: A handbook of psychological treatment approaches.* New York: Pergamon Press.

Corah, N.L., Gale, E.N., & Illig, S.J. (1979). The use of relaxation and distraction to reduce psychological stress during dental procedures. *Journal of the American Dental Association, 98,* 390–394.

Cousins, N. (1989). *Head first: The biology of hope.* New York: E.P. Dutton.

Cotanch, P.H. (1983). Relaxation training for control of nausea and vomiting in patients receiving chemotherapy. *Cancer Nursing, 6,* 277–283.

Cotanch, P.H., Hockenberry, M., & Herman, S. (1985). Self-hypnosis, antiemetic therapy in children receiving chemotherapy. *Oncology Nursing Forum, 12,* 41–46.

Cotanch, P.H., & Strum, S. (1987). Progressive muscle relaxation as antiemetic therapy for cancer patients. *Oncology Nursing Forum, 14,* 33–37.

Crasilneck, H.B., & Hall, J.A. (1975). *Clinical hypnosis: Principles and applications.* New York: Grune & Stratton.

Dahlquist, L.M., Gil, K.M., Armstrong, F.D., Ginsberg, A., & Jones, B. (1985). Behavioral management of children's distress during chemotherapy. *Journal of Behavior Therapy and Experimental Psychiatry, 16,* 325–329.

Daut, R.L., Cleeland, C.S., & Flannery, R.C. (1983). Development of the Wisconsin brief pain questionnaire to assess pain in cancer and other diseases. *Pain, 17,* 197–210.

DeBetz, B., & Sunnen, G. (1985). *A primer of clinical hypnosis.* Littleton, MA: PSG Publishing Co.

Dolgin, M., Katz, E., McGinty, K., & Siegel, S. (1985). Anticipatory nausea and vomiting in pediatric cancer patients. *Pediatrics, 75,* 547–552.

Dryden, W., & Golden, W.L. (1986). *Cognitive-behavioural approaches to psychotherapy.* London: Harper & Row.

Dunn, R.J. (1979). Cognitive modification with depression-prone psychiatric patients. *Cognitive Therapy and Research, 3,* 307–317.

D'Zurilla, T.J., & Goldfried, M.R. (1971). Problem solving and behavior modification. *Journal of Abnormal Psychology, 78,* 107–126.

Elliott, C.H., & Olson, R.A. (1983). The management of children's distress in response to painful medical treatment for burn injuries. *Behaviour Research and Therapy, 21,* 675–683.

Elliott, C.H., & Ozolins, M. (1983). Imagery and imagination in the treatment of children. In C.L. Walker & M. Roberts (Eds.), *Handbook of clinical child psychology.* Homewood, IL: Dorsey Press.

Ellis, A. (1962). *Reason and emotion in psychotherapy.* New York: Lyle Stuart.

Ellis, A., & Harper, R.A. (1975). *A new guide to rational living.* North Hollywood, CA: Wilshire.

Erickson, M.H. (1959). Hypnosis in painful terminal illness. *American Journal of Clinical Hypnosis, 1,* 117–121.

Erickson, M.H. (1966). The interspersal hypnotic technique for symptom correction and pain control. *American Journal of Clinical Hypnosis, 8,* 198–209.

Erickson, M.H. (1983). *Healing in hypnosis: The seminars, workshops, and lectures of Milton H. Erickson: Vol. 1.* New York: Irvington.

Farthing, G.W., Venturino, M., & Brown, S.W. (1984). Suggestion and distraction in the control of pain: Test of two hypotheses. *Journal of Abnormal Psychology, 93,* 266–276.

Fensterheim, H., & Baer, J. (1975). *Don't say yes when you want to say no.* New York: David Mckay.

Ferster, C.B. (1973). A functional analysis of depression. *American Psychologist, 28,* 857–870.

Foley, K.M. (1979). Pain syndromes in patients with cancer. In J.J. Bonica & V. Ventafredda (Eds.), *Advances in pain research and therapy: Vol. 2.* New York: Raven Press.

Foley, K.M. (1986). The treatment of pain in the patient with cancer. *Cancer — A Cancer Journal for Clinicians, 36* (4), 194–215.

Fordyce, W.E. (1976). Behavioral concepts in chronic pain in illness. In P.O. Davidson (Ed.), *The behavior management of anxiety, depression, and pain.* New York: Brunner/Mazel.

Gardner, G.G., & Olness, K. (1981). *Hypnosis and hypnotherapy with children.* New York: Grune & Stratton.

Golden, W.L. (1983a). Rational-Emotive hypnotherapy: Principles and techniques. *British Journal of Cognitive Psychotherapy, 1*(1), 47–56.

Golden, W.L. (1983b). Resistance in cognitive-behaviour therapy. *British Journal of Cognitive Psychotherapy, 1*(2), 33–42.

Golden, W.L. (1985). Commonalities between cognitive-behavior therapy and hypnotherapy. *The Cognitive Behaviorist, 7,* 2–4.

Golden, W.L. (1986). An integration of Ericksonian and cognitive-behavioral hypnotherapy in the treatment of anxiety disorder. In E.T. Dowd & J.M. Healy (Eds.), *Case studies in hypnotherapy.* New York: Guilford Press.

Golden, W.L., Dowd, E.T., & Friedberg, F. (1987). *Hypnotherapy: A modern approach.* New York: Pergamon Press.

Golden, W.L., & Dryden, W. (1986). Cognitive-behavioural therapies: Commonalities, divergences and future development. In W. Dryden & W.L. Golden (Eds.), *Cognitive-behavioural approaches to psychotherapy.* London: Harper & Row.

Golden, W.L., & Friedberg, F. (1986). Cognitive-behavioural hypnotherapy. In W. Dryden & W.L. Golden (Eds.), *Cognitive-behavioural approaches to psychotherapy.* London: Harper & Row.

Goldfried, M.R. (1971). Systematic desensitization as training in self-control. *Journal of Consulting and Clinical Psychology, 37,* 228–234.

Goldfried, M.R., & Davison, G.C. (1976). *Clinical behavior therapy.* New York: Holt, Rinehart & Winston.

Goldstein, A. (1973). Are opiate tolerance and dependence reversible: Implications for the treatment of heroin addiction. In H. Capple & A. Le Blanc (Eds.), *Biological and behavioral approaches to drug dependence.* Toronto: Addiction Research Foundation.

Greer, S. (1988). Measuring mental adjustment to cancer. In M. Watson, S. Greer, & C. Thomas (Eds.), *Psychosocial oncology.* Oxford: Pergamon Press.

Grossarth-Maticek, R., Bastiaans, J., & Kanazir, D.T. (1985). Psychosocial factors as strong predictors of mortality from cancer, ischemic heart disease and stroke: The Yugoslav prospective study. *Journal of Psychosomatic Research, 29,* 167–176.

Grossarth-Maticek, R., Schmidt, P., Vetter, H., & Arndt, S. (1984). Psychotherapy research in oncology. In A. Steptoe and A. Mathews (Eds.), *Health care and human behavior.* London: Academic Press.

Grossarth-Maticek, R., Siegrest, J., & Vetter, H. (1982). Interpersonal repression as a predictor of cancer. *Social Science and Medicine, 16,* 493–498.

Gruber, B.L., Hall, N.R., Hersh, S.P., & Dubois, P. (1988). Immune system and psychologic changes in metastic cancer patients while using ritualized relaxation and guided imagery: A pilot study. *Scandinavian Journal of Behavior Therapy, 17,* 25–46.

Hailey, B.J., & White, J.G. (1983). Systematic desensitization for anticipatory nausea associated with chemotherapy. *Psychosomatic, 24,* 289–292.

Hammond, D. (1982). Multidisciplinary management of childhood cancers: A model for the future. In M. Willoughby & S.E. Siegel (Eds.), *Hematology and oncology* (pp. 1–13). London: Butterworth Scientific.

Hauck, P.A. (1966). The neurotic agreement in psychotherapy. *Rational Living, 1,* 31–34.

Hauck, P.A. (1976). *Overcoming depression.* Philadelphia: Westminster Press.

Hendler, C.S., & Redd, W.H. (1986). Fear of hypnosis: The role of labeling in patients' acceptance of behavioral intervention. *Behavior Therapy, 17,* 2–13.

Hilgard, E.R. (1979). Divided consciousness in hypnosis: The implications of the hidden observer. In E. Fromm & R.E. Shor (Eds.), *Hypnosis: Developments in research and new perspectives* (pp. 45–79). New York: Aldine.

Hilgard, E.R., & Hilgard, J. (1975). *Hypnosis in the relief of pain.* Los Altos, CA: Kaufman.

Hilgard, E.R., & LeBaron, S. (1982). Relief of anxiety and pain in children and adolescents with cancer: Quantitative measures and clinical observations. *International Journal of Clinical and Experimental Hypnosis, 30,* 417–442.

Hilgard, J.R., & LeBaron, S. (1984). *Hypnotherapy of pain in children with cancer.* Los Altos, CA: Kaufman.

Hockenberry, M.J., & Bologna-Vaughn, S. (1985). Preparation for intrusive procedures using noninvasive techniques in children with cancer: State of the art vs. new trends. *Cancer Nursing, 8,* 97–102.

Hoffman, I., & Futterman, E.H. (1971). Coping with waiting: psychiatric intervention and study in the waiting room of a pediatric oncology clinic. *Comprehensive Psychiatry, 12,* 67–81.

International Association for the Study of Pain. (1979). Subcommittee on taxonomy pain terms: A list with definitions and notes on usage. *Pain, 6,* 249–252.

Jacobson, E. (1938). *Progressive relaxation.* Chicago: University of Chicago.

Jay, S.M., & Elliott, C. H. (1984). Behavioral observation scales for measuring children's distress: The effects of increased methodological rigor. *Journal of Consulting and Clinical Psychology, 52,* 1106–1107.

Jay, S.M., Elliott, C.H., Katz, E., & Siegel, S.E. (1987). Cognitive-behavioral and pharmacologic interventions for children's distress during painful medical procedures. *Journal of Consulting and Clinical Psychology, 55,* 860–865.

Jay, S.M., Elliott, C.H., Ozolins, M., Olson, R.A., & Pruitt, S.D. (1985). Behavioral management of children's distress during painful medical procedures. *Behaviour Research and Therapy, 23,* 513–520.

Jay, S.M., Elliott, C., & Varni, J.W. (1986). Acute and chronic pain in adults and children with cancer. *Journal of Consulting and Clinical Psychology, 54,* 601–607.

Jay, S.M., Ozolins, M., Elliott, C.H., & Caldwell, S. (1983). Assessment of children's distress during painful medical procedures. *Health Psychology, 2,* 133–147.

Katz, E.R., Kellerman, J., & Siegel, S. (1980). Behavioral distress in children with cancer undergoing medical procedures: Developmental considerations. *Journal of Consulting and Clinical Psychology, 48,* 356–365.

Katz, E.R., Kellerman, J., & Siegel, S.E. (1981). Anxiety as an affective focus in the clinical study of acute behavioral distress: A reply to Schacham and Daut. *Journal of Consulting and Clinical Psychology, 49,* 470–471.

Kellerman, J., Zeltzer, L.K., Ellenberg, I., & Dash, J. (1983). Adolescents with cancer: Hypnosis for the reduction of acute pain associated with medical procedures. *Journal of Adolescent Health Care, 4,* 85–90.

Kneier, A.W., & Temoshok, L. (1984). Repressive coping reactions in patients with malignant melanoma as compared to cardiovascular disease patients. *Journal of Psychosomatic Research, 28,* 145–155.

Kolko, D.J., & Rickard-Figueroa, J.L. (1985). Effects of video games on the adverse corollaries of chemotherapy in pediatric oncology patients: A single-case analysis. *Journal of Consulting and Clinical Psychology, 53,* 223–228.

Kozier, B., & Lea, G. (1979). *Fundamentals of nursing: Concepts and procedures.* Menlo Park, CA: Addison-Wesley.

Kübler-Ross, E. (1969). *On death and dying.* New York: Macmillan.

LaBaw, W., Holton, C., Tewell, K., & Eccles, D. (1975). The use of self-hypnosis by children with cancer. *American Journal of Clinical Hypnosis, 17,* 233–238.

Lange, A.J., & Jakubowski, P. (1976). *Responsible assertive behavior.* Champaign, IL: Research Press.

Lansdown, R., & Goldman, A. (1988). Annotation: The psychological care of children with malignant disease. *Journal of Child Psychology and Psychiatry, 5,* 555–567.

Lansky, S.B., & Gendel, M. (1978). Symbiotic regressive behavior patterns in childhood malignancy. *Clinical Pediatrics, 17,* 133–138.

Lascari, A.D., & Stehbens, J.A. (1973). The reactions of families to childhood leukemia. *Clinical Pediatrics, 12,* 210–214.

Lazarus, A.A. (1967). In support of technical eclecticism. *Psychological Reports, 21,* 415–416.

Lazarus, A.A. (1968). Learning theory and the treatment of depression. *Behaviour Research and Therapy, 6,* 83–89.

Lazarus, A.A. (1973). "Hypnosis" as a facilitator in behavior therapy. *International Journal of Clinical and Experimental Hypnosis, 21,* 25–31.

Lazarus, A.A. (1981). *The practice of multimodal therapy.* New York: McGraw-Hill.

Lazarus, A.A., & Abramovitz, A. (1962). The use of "emotive imagery" in the treatment of children's phobias. *Journal of Mental Science, 108,* 191–195.

Lea, P., Ware, P., & Monroe, R. (1960). The hypnotic control of intractable pain. *American Journal of Clinical Hypnosis, 3,* 3–8.

LeBaron, S., & Zeltzer, L.K. (1984). Behavioral intervention for reducing chemotherapy-related nausea and vomiting in adolescents with cancer. *Journal of Adolescent Health Care, 5,* 178–182.

Le Shan, L. (1977). *You can fight for your life.* New York: Evans.

Levine, A.S., & Hersh, S.P. (1982). The psychosocial concomitants of cancer in young patients. In A.S. Levine (Ed.), *Cancer in the young.* New York: Masson.

Lewinsohn, P.M. (1974). A behavioral approach to depression. In R.M. Friedman & M.M. Katz (Eds.), *The psychology of depression: Contemporary theory and research*. New York: John Wiley & Sons.

Lyles, J.N., Burish, T.G., Krozely, M.G., & Oldham, R.K. (1982). Efficacy of relaxation training and guided imagery in reducing the aversiveness of cancer chemotherapy. *Journal of Consulting and Clinical Psychology, 50*, 509–524.

Maguire, P., Comaroff, J., Ramsell, P.J., & Morris-Jones, P.H. (1979). Psychological and social problems in families of children with leukemia. In P.H. Morris-Jones (Ed.), *Topics in pediatrics: I. Hematology and oncology*. Turnbridge Wells: Pitman Medical.

Margolis, C.G. (1983). Hypnotic imagery with cancer patients. *American Journal of Clinical Hypnosis, 25*, 128–134.

Margolis, C.G. (1986). Special pain problems. In E.T. Dowd & J.M. Healy (Eds.), *Case studies in hypnotherapy*. New York: Guilford Press.

Marks, R.M., & Sacher, E.J. (1973). Undertreatment of medical inpatients with narcotic analgesics. *Annals of Internal Medicine, 78*, 173–181.

McCaul, K.D., & Malott, J.M. (1984). Distraction and coping with pain. *Psychological Bulletin, 95*, 516–533.

Meichenbaum, D. (1971). Examination of model characteristics in reducing avoidance behavior. *Journal of Personality and Social Psychology, 17*, 298–307.

Meichenbaum, D. (1977). *Cognitive-behavior modification: An integrative approach*. New York: Plenum Publishing.

Meichenbaum, D. (1985). *Stress inoculation training*. New York: Pergamon Press.

Melamed, B.G., & Siegel, L.J. (1975). Reduction of anxiety in children facing hospitalization and surgery by use of filmed modeling. *Journal of Consulting and Clinical Psychology, 43*, 511–521.

Melzack, R. (1975). The McGill Pain Questionnaire: Major properties and scoring methods. *Pain, 1*, 277–299.

Melzack, R., & Wall, P.D. (1965). Pain mechanisms: A new theory. *Science, 150*, 971–979.

Minuchin, S. (1974). *Families and family therapy*. Cambridge, MA: University Press.

Morrisey, J.R. (1963). Children's adaptation to fatal illness. *Social Work, 8*, 81–88.

Morris-Jones, P.H. (1987). Advances in managing childhood cancer. *British Medical Journal, 245*, 4–6.

Morrow, G.R. (1982). Prevalence and correlates of anticipatory nausea and vomiting in chemotherapy patients. *Journal of the National Cancer Institute, 68*, 484–488.

Morrow, G.R. (1986). Effect of the cognitive hierarchy in the systematic desensitization treatment of anticipatory nausea in cancer patients: A component comparison with relaxation only, counseling and no treatment. *Cognitive Therapy and Research, 10*, 421–446.

Morrow, G.R., & Morrell, C. (1982). Behavioral treatment for the anticipatory nausea and vomiting induced by cancer chemotherapy. *New England Journal of Medicine, 307*, 1476–1480.

Natterson, J.M., & Knudson, A.G. (1960). Observations concerning fear of death in fatally ill children and their mothers. *Psychosomatic Medicine, 22*, 456–465.

Nesse, R.M., Carli, T., Curtis, G.C., & Kleinman, P.D. (1980). Pretreatment nausea in cancer chemotherapy. *Psychosomatic Medicine, 42*, 33–36.

Nocella, J., & Kaplan, B.M. (1982). Training children to cope with dental treatment. *Journal of Pediatric Psychology, 7*, 175–178.

Novaco, R. (1975). *Anger control: The development and evaluation of an experimental treatment*. Lexington, MA: Heath.

Olness, K. (1981). Imagery (self-hypnosis) as adjunct therapy in childhood cancer: Clinical experience with 25 patients. *Journal of Pediatric Hematology/Oncology, 3*, 313–321.

Persky, V.W., Kempthorne-Rawson, J., & Shekelle, R.B. (1987). Personality and risk of cancer: 20-year follow-up of the Western Electric study. *Psychosomatic Medicine, 49,* 435–449.

Peterson, L., & Shigetomi, C. (1981). The use of coping techniques to minimize anxiety in hospitalized children. *Behavior Therapy, 12,* 1–14.

Redd, W.H. (1982). Treatment of excessive crying in a terminal cancer patient: A time-series analysis. *Journal of Behavioral Medicine, 5,* 225–235.

Redd, W.H. (1988). Behavioral approaches to treatment-related distress. *Cancer: A Cancer Journal for Clinicians, 38,* 138–144.

Redd, W.H., Andersen, G.V., & Minagawa, R.Y. (1982). Hypnotic control of anticipatory emesis in patients receiving cancer chemotherapy. *Journal of Consulting and Clinical Psychology, 50,* 14–19.

Redd, W.H., Jacobsen, P.B., Die-Trill, M., Dermatis, H., McEvoy, M., & Holland, J.C. (1987). Cognitive/attentional distraction in the control of conditioned nausea in pediatric cancer patients receiving chemotherapy. *Journal of Consulting and Clinical Psychology, 55,* 391–395.

Rosenbaum, E.H., & Rosenbaum, I.R. (1980). *A comprehensive guide for cancer patients and their families.* Palo Alto, CA: Bull Publishing.

Rush, A.J., Beck, A.T., Kovacs, M., & Hollon, S. (1977). Comparative efficacy of cognitive therapy and pharmacotherapy in the treatment of depressed outpatients. *Cognitive Therapy and Research, 1,* 17–37.

Sacerdote, P. (1962). The place of hypnosis in the relief of severe protracted pain. *American Journal of Clinical Hypnosis, 4,* 150–157.

Sacerdote, P. (1970). Theory and practice of pain control in malignancy and other protracted or recurring illnesses. *International Journal of Clinical and Experimental Hypnosis, 18,* 160–180.

Salter, A. (1941). Three techniques of autohypnosis. *Journal of General Psychology, 24,* 423–438.

Sanders, S. (1979). Behavioral assessment and treatment of clinical pain: Appraisal and current status. In M. Hersen, R.M. Eisler, & P.M. Miller (Eds.), *Progress in behavior modification* (pp. 249–291). New York: Academic Press.

Schacham, S., & Daut, R. (1981). Anxiety or pain: What does the scale measure? *Journal of Consulting and Clinical Psychology, 49,* 468–469.

Scheng, H., & Blohmke, M. (1988). Associations between selected life events and cancer. *Behavioral Medicine, 14,* 119–124.

Shapiro, A. (1983). Psychotherapy as adjunct treatment for cancer patients. *American Journal of Clinical Hypnosis, 25,* 150–155.

Shekelle, R.B., Raynor, W.J., & Ostfeld, A.M. (1981). Psychological depression and 17-year risk of death from cancer. *Psychosomatic Medicine, 43,* 117–125.

Siegel, B.S. (1986). *Love, medicine & miracles.* New York: Harper & Row.

Siegel, L., & Peterson, L. (1980). Stress reduction in young dental patients through coping skills and sensory information. *Journal of Consulting and Clinical Psychology, 48,* 785–787.

Simonton, S., Simonton, O.C., & Creighton, J.L. (1978). *Getting well again.* New York: Bantam Books.

Spanos, N.P., & Barber, T.X. (1974). Toward a convergence in hypnosis research. *American Psychologist, 29,* 500–511.

Spanos, N.P., & Barber, T.X. (1976). Behavior modification and hypnosis. In M. Hersen, R.M. Eisler, & P.M. Miller (Eds.), *Progress in behavior modification.* New York: Academic Press.

Spanos, N.P., Radtke-Bodorik, H.L., Ferguson, J.D., & Jones, B. (1979). The effects of hypnotic susceptibility, suggestions for analgesia, and the utilization of cognitive strategies on the reduction of pain. *Journal of Abnormal Psychology, 88,* 282–292.

Spiegel, D. (1985). The use of hypnosis in controlling cancer pain. *Cancer: A Cancer Journal for Clinicians, 35,* 221–231.

Spiegel, D., & Bloom,, J.R. (1983). Group therapy and hypnosis reduce metastatic breast carcinoma pain. *Psychosomatic Medicine, 45,* 333–339.

Spiegel, D., Bloom, J.R., Kraemer, H.C., & Gottheil, E. (1989). Effect of psychosocial treatment on survival of patients with metastatic breast cancer. *The Lancet, 9,* 888–891.

Spinetta, J.J., & Maloney, L.J. (1975). Death anxiety in the outpatient leukemic child. *Pediatrics, 56,* 1034–1037.

Spivack, G., Platt, J.J., & Shure, M.B. (1976). *The problem solving approach to adjustment.* San Francisco: Jossey-Bass.

Tan, S. (1982). Cognitive and cognitive-behavioral methods for pain control: A selective review. *Pain, 12,* 201–228.

Teichman, Y. (1984). Cognitive family therapy. *British Journal of Cognitive Psychotherapy, 2,* 1–10.

Temoshok, L., Heller, B.W., Sagebiel, R.W., Blois, M.S., Sweet, D.M., DiClemente, R.J., & Gold, M.L. (1985). The relationship of psychosocial factors to prognostic indicators in cutaneous malignant melanoma. *Journal of Psychosomatic Research, 29,* 139–153.

Turk, D., Meichenbaum, D., & Genest, M. (1983). *Pain and behavioral medicine.* New York: Guilford Press.

Turner, J.A., & Chapman, C.R. (1982). Psychological interventions for chronic pain: A critical review. II: Operant conditioning, hypnosis, and cognitive-behavioral therapy. *Pain, 12,* 23–46.

Van Dongen-Melman, J.E.W.M., & Sanders-Woudstra, J.A.R. (1986). Psychosocial aspects of childhood cancer: A review of the literature. *Journal of Child Psychology and Psychiatry, 27,* 145–180.

Welch-McCaffrey, D. (1983). When it comes to cancer, think family. *Nursing, 13,* 32–35.

West, B.L., & Piccionne, C. (1982). Cognitive-behavioral techniques in treating anorexia and depression in a cancer patient. *The Behavior Therapist, 5,* 115–117.

Winiarski, M.G. (1991). *AIDS-related psychotherapy.* New York: Pergamon Press.

Wolpe, J. (1958). *Psychotherapy by reciprocal inhibition.* Stanford, CA: Stanford University.

Zeltzer, L.K. (1980). The adolescent with cancer. In J. Kellerman (Ed.), *Psychological aspects of childhood cancer.* Springfield, IL: Charles C. Thomas.

Zeltzer, L.K., Kellerman, J., Ellenberg, L., Barbour, J.S., Dash, J., & Rigler, D. (1980). Self-hypnosis for reduction of pain and anxiety in adolescents with cancer. *Pediatric Research, 14,* 430.

Zeltzer, L.K., Kellerman, J., Ellenberg, L., & Dash, J. (1983). Hypnosis for reduction of vomiting associated with chemotherapy and disease in adolescents with cancer. *Journal of Adolescent Health Care, 4,* 77–84.

Zeltzer, L.K., & LeBaron, S. (1982). Hypnosis and nonhypnotic techniques for reduction of pain and anxiety during painful procedures in children and adolescents with cancer. *Journal of Pediatrics, 101,* 1032–1035.

Zeltzer, L.K., LeBaron, S., & Zeltzer, P. (1984). The effectiveness of behavioral intervention for reducing nausea and vomiting in children receiving chemotherapy. *Journal of Clinical Oncology, 2,* 683–690.

Zonderman, A.B., Costa, P.T., & McCrae, R.R. (1989). Depression as a risk for cancer morbidity and mortality in a nationally representative sample. *Journal of the American Medical Association, 262* (9), 1191–1195.

Author Index

Subject Index

About the Authors

William L. Golden is on the faculty of Cornell Medical College, the Institute for Rational-Emotive Therapy in New York City, and the Institute for Behavior Therapy in New York City. He is on the editorial boards of the *Journal of Cognitive Psychotherapy: An International Quarterly* and the *Journal of Rational-Emotive and Cognitive-Behavior Therapy.* Dr. Golden has written extensively on cognitive-behavior therapy and hypnosis. He has a private practice in New York City and Briarcliff Manor, N.Y. (Westchester County). He is a member of the American Psychological Association, the Association for the Advancement of Behavior Therapy, and the Westchester County Psychological Association.

Wayne D. Gersh is the codirector of the Westchester Center for Behavior Therapy and is engaged in full-time private practice. He is on the staff of the crisis counseling team for the Westchester Division of The American Cancer Society. In addition, he has developed programs for working with cancer patients and their families. He is a member of the American Psychological Association, the Association for the Advancement of Behavior Therapy, and the Westchester County Psychological Association.

David M. Robbins is the codirector of the Westchester Center for Behavior Therapy, where he directs the treatment program for children with behavioral and social problems. He has also developed several programs for helping children cope with cancer and leukemia. He is a member of the American Psychological Association, the Association for the Advancement of Behavior Therapy, and the Westchester County Psychological Association.

Psychology Practitioner Guidebooks

Editors
Arnold P. Goldstein, Syracuse University
Leonard Krasner, Stanford University & SUNY at Stony Brook
Sol L. Garfield, Washington University in St. Louis